JOGGING WITH LYDIARD

Books by Arthur Lydiard & Garth Gilmour:
RUN TO THE TOP
RUN FOR YOUR LIFE
RUN THE LYDIARD WAY
RUNNING WITH LYDIARD

Other books by Garth Gilmour:
A CLEAN PAIR OF HEELS (with
Murray Halberg)
NO BUGLES, NO DRUMS (with
Peter Snell)
DARDIR ON SQUASH (with
Dardir el Bakary)
NO GRASS BETWEEN MY TOES
(with Eve Rimmer)

JOGGING WITH LYDIARD

Arthur Lydiard
with
Garth Gilmour

HODDER AND STOUGHTON
AUCKLAND LONDON SYDNEY TORONTO

Typeset by Glenfield Graphics Ltd, Auckland.
Printed and bound in Hong Kong for Hodder and Stoughton
Ltd, View Road, Glenfield, Auckland, New Zealand.

Contents

Introduction

W HEN 20 ODDLY assorted New Zealanders gathered in an Auckland city park one Sunday morning 21 years ago to listen to and have a preliminary jog with Arthur Lydiard, jogging as an integral part of the life pattern of millions of modern men and women was born. The speed with which it has captured people's imagination around the world and stirred them into physical action is one of the wonders of our age.

By today's yardsticks, it was a pathetic little meeting in 1961 — about as insignificant as the button you would push to fire a nuclear device. The mushroom cloud of jogging which it triggered has been expanding around and enveloping the world ever since. The 20 bloomed into hundreds, then thousands and now millions. Their beginning appears to have no ending.

What began as a tentative individual exercise for a few has become a movement of international vitality, often with national backing and sponsorship. East Germany's State-organised 'Run For Your Life' programme was inspired by and took its name from Arthur Lydiard's second book, published in 1965.

The fun runs, like the sponsored Round-the-Bays run in Auckland, which this year (1982) attracted an estimated 80,000 people to run together over a 12-kilometre course, are a direct sequel because the jogging boom became a commercial bonanza for the makers of running shoes, running clothing, running aids and medications and it became vital for them to organise people together to keep the promotion of jogging in the forefront of attention.

The reasons for jogging's survival and continuing growth through two decades while all manner of other fads have come and gone are few but inarguable. Even the critics have been forced to accept that people are healthier and, usually, happier through jogging; it is perhaps one of the cheapest and most convenient recreations — a good pair of shoes and any old comfortable and lightweight running gear is adequate, you can do it alone or in a crowd, morning, noon or night, regardless of the weather or where you are.

Arthur Lydiard, who became an overnight coaching success with his preparation of Peter Snell, Murray Halberg and Barry Magee to win medals for New Zealand at the 1960 Rome Olympics and then, with a handful of others, to dominate middle and distance racing all round the world, has since become the globe-trotting prophet of jogging. No-one in history has acquired more disciples without actively seeking them or using force or coercion. He is the confidant of and consultant to physiologists, coaches and sports medicine experts in many countries and, probably, the biggest single factor in the physical fitness revolution which has swept most of the western nations and much of the rest of the world in recent years.

Virtually every man, woman, youth and child who jogs for fitness does so because Arthur Lydiard took running for fun, relaxation and a happier way of life out of the pre-1960s realm of something only odd ex-athletes did, into a new era of understanding and desire for a fuller enjoyment of life.

Golfers, swimmers, footballers, squash players, tennis players — particularly those at the top of their sport — have adopted it as an essential adjunct to the normal playing skills they practise. A very high percentage of the world's athletes now train exactly to, or to close imitations of, the Lydiard system.

Not all joggers know that Arthur Lydiard's original inspiration is what they are following but, however indirectly they received the message, it is. Through his training of Snell, Halberg, Magee and company, Lydiard revolutionised the competitive running world, overturning traditional techniques and beliefs wherever runners run and coaches coach and, together, look for better performance.

Through his preaching of the gentler art of jogging, he has also revolutionised the approach to the grace of growing old without growing old. Less than two decades ago, the over-50 entrant in a footrace was regarded, however kindly, as slightly touched in the head; today, many distance races, particularly marathons, are numerically dominated by veterans. Veterans' track and field contests at all levels up to international are commonplace. The early morning and evening street scenes in thousands of towns and cities are enlivened by people running because it makes them feel better, enjoy other leisure pursuits more, work more efficiently and more totally enjoy the rewards of being alive. Business executive or labourer, student or salesman, housewife or office typist, career woman or mother, they all jog for their lives.

This book is Arthur Lydiard's philosophy of jogging, just as it was 21 years ago. It is your guide to why you should jog, if you are not jogging already; how you jog, or jog better if you are already; how it holds back the degeneration that does not necessarily have to accompany the advancing years. The message has not altered because the only change has been the flashfire spread and acceptance of jogging into an international cult.

In a foreword to *Run For Your Life*, Dr Norrie Jefferson, president of the New Zealand Foundation of Sports Medicine, said: 'The fact that the theories behind many of the results of these very practical experiments (in jogging) are still being confirmed by medical research workers speaks volumes for the breadth of vision and tenacity of purpose of Arthur Lydiard ... I am convinced that if the jogging system of exercise for the human body does nothing else but increase our resistance to illness and disease, it has helped to attain a very worthy objective in preventive and social medicine.'

The confirmation and proof by the experts has continued since then, but perhaps the most important proof has been supplied by the countless millions who climb so regularly into their running shoes and take to the streets, roads, beaches, parks and forest trails of the world for a gentle jog for their lives.

Garth Gilmour
Auckland, 1982

1. Your heart at work

J OGGING IS AN affair of the heart. Just as you do, it begins with the heart and it ends there. All other benefits are subsidiary to the exercise and development of a heart that will continue to beat steadily, strongly and easily to supply the rest of you with healthy, well-toned blood.

Let's look at how it works because you need to understand what it does and how it can go wrong before you begin to do anything for it.

The principles behind the circulation of the blood, which is the heart's function, are almost ridiculously simple. No more complicated than some hot-water systems and no different from all those other muscles in our bodies of which we are so much more conscious and to which we normally pay much more attention. More than one person has worked diligently at making the biceps muscles bulge while the heart muscle atrophies.

Like many simple truths, it took mankind a long time to learn about the heart. Philosophers and scientists spent about the first 1600 years of Christianity arguing about the heart and its importance in the body. Most upheld the astonishing notion that the liver, not the heart, was the main organ of blood circulation and that the heart only added air which it received from the lungs. It was believed that the blood ebbed back and forth in the arteries and veins. One mediaeval scientist who disputed this concept was burned at the stake.

Then, about 1600, England's William Harvey proclaimed a new truth: The heart was, in fact, a pump, forcing blood via the arteries into the tissues, from where it returned through the veins to the heart, was pumped on to the lungs to pick up oxygen and then returned for recirculation to the tissues. It did not, said Harvey, ebb to and fro — and he was the first person to say so and get away with it. His research into the functions of the heart remains one of the fantastic feats of the human intellect. He explained that, in the tissues of the body, the blood must percolate through channels so fine that the human eye could not see them and that they formed a direct link between the arteries and the veins. He reached this conclusion by sheer logic and died four years before the invention of the microscope which confirmed that these channels, now called capillaries, did exist and did do the job he claimed for them.

Tissues need oxygen to spark the chemical reactions which provide energy just as a fire needs oxygen before it will burn and generate heat. The blood's important function is to carry that oxygen to the tissues. It is first picked up from the air in the lungs. The oxygen-enriched blood (reddish in colour) travels to the heart and is pumped to the tissues where the oxygen content is extracted. The oxygen-depleted blood (bluish in colour) then returns to the heart to be pumped back to the lungs for re-oxygenation.

The heart, therefore, is receiving and transferring two types of blood at once — enriched from the lungs and depleted from the tissues. To keep these two streams apart, the heart chamber is divided in two by a muscular partition called the septum. A partially deficient septum, which allows the two types of blood to mix to some extent, is one of the common types of congenital defect in humans — the well-known 'hole in the heart'.

The left and right chambers formed by the septum are further divided into two parts — the auricle, which has a thin wall, has little pumping action and serves mainly as a reservoir; and the ventricle, which has a thick muscular wall and does the main pumping.

The veins which deliver the blood from the tissues are called venae cavae and drain into the right auricle. Veins bringing the blood from the lungs are called pulmonary veins and empty into the left auricle. From the right auricle, blood passes into the right ventricle, which pumps it into the lungs through the pulmonary arteries. Blood from the left auricle, passed into the left ventricle, is pumped to the tissues through a large artery called the aorta.

The efficiency of any pump depends on a valve which allows the fluid being pumped to flow in the desired direction. If the valve leaks, the pump has to do more work to compensate for the leakage. The heart, being the super-efficient organ it is, has four sets of valves. The first two are at the opening between each auricle and ventricle and allow blood to flow only from auricle to ventricle. When the ventricle contracts, these valves close and the blood cannot normally escape back into the auricle. When the ventricles relax, the valves open again and allow blood through from the auricles to refill the ventricles.

Ventricle outflow is controlled by the other valves to the aorta and the pulmonary arteries and prevents leakage back into the ventricles when they are relaxed for refilling. Rheumatic fever and some other diseases can damage these heart valves so that leaks occur.

Like any other good pump, the heart is made to vary its output. In a resting person, it beats between 65 and 80 times a minute and copes in that time with about seven pints (four litres) of blood. This volume, called cardiac output, can be increased, with exercise, as much as six to ten times.

The heart's contraction phase, when blood is being expelled, is called systole. The relaxation phase — outflow valves shut, inflow valves open — is diastole. During diastole, the heart passively fills like a reservoir and the heart muscle is relaxed and going through chemical changes which recharge the sources of energy used up in the preceding systole. If the heart beat is quickened, the diastole period is shortened and the process of recharging may be impeded.

A sound heart, like a sound car, can be driven far and fast without harm but periods of rest and recovery are needed. As we age, this need generally increases — but not as much as people imagine. Like the sound car, regular maintenance and sensible use can keep the heart functioning, like a vintage

13

vehicle, in as-new condition.

An increase in heart size is interpreted and accepted now as a normal physiological adaptation to sound training and there is no evidence to show that hard endurance training can harm a healthy heart. In fact, some endurance work is now known to be important in many cases as part of the treatment for coronary occlusion, which we discuss shortly.

It has been demonstrated, too, that the trained person can perform more work before reaching maximum heart rate than the untrained person. This is an underlying principle of the Lydiard system of marathon-type or endurance training for athletes — and of controlled sensible jogging.

In the average person, the cardiac output or minute volume of the heart — the amount of blood pumped through every 60 seconds — rises during exercise from seven to 35 pints (four to 20 litres). In the well-trained person, it can rise to 70 pints (40 litres). This increase depends on stroke volume — the amount of blood pumped at each beat — as well as the pulse or beat rate. Stroke volume increases as the pulse rate increases and the limit is reached when the pulse rate becomes so high that the heart does not have time to refill adequately. The stroke volume then decreases. The trained or fit person takes longer to reach this limit.

Increased arterial pressure and better diastolic filling help the increased stroke volume. For a standard amount of work, the heart rate becomes slower as training progresses and these changes mean a decreasing load on the cardio-vascular system and indicate the adaption to the demands of exercise.

Women show the same reactions to hard training as men, though they can be affected by menstruation.

The pulse, which runners and joggers who know their normal at-rest rate when they begin training can use as a simple measure of their standard of fitness, is simply explained. Each time the heart beats, it pumps blood into the arteries; the arterial wall just beyond the heart outflow valve expands to accommodate the added blood volume and this expansion travels through the arteries like the ripple from a stone tossed in still water. You feel that expansion wave when you take your pulse.

2. Heart murmurs and malfunctions

A S WE'VE SAID, the pulse at rest varies in rate from 65 to 80 beats a minute but is influenced by many factors, mainly exercise, nervousness, temperature, excitement and fever. Normal or stimulated, the rate is fairly regular. Irregularities that do occur are mostly due to added beats called extra systole. These may cause the feeling that the heart is thumping, missing beats or even momentarily pausing — all sensations which can lead people to think they have heart trouble. Only 50 years ago, many doctors would have agreed with this lay verdict and condemned many people, without justification, to lives of cardiac invalidism.

The great English practitioner, James McKenzie, first discovered and taught that these palpitations were not usually due to heart disease at all. McKenzie, in fact, launched the great era of cardiology, fighting hard to make doctors and patients alike realise that heart disease is too readily confused with symptoms produced by nervousness and fatigue, and that true heart disease sufferers were generally being advised to restrict their activities too much.

Normally, the arterial walls expand and contract each time the heart forces blood into them. With increasing age, some of the elasticity is lost and the arterial wall becomes harder, mainly due to the replacement of the elastic tissues by a more rigid substance. This happens to most of us sooner or later but, because it doesn't obstruct the flow of blood, it rarely causes concern. It is a condition which must be distinguished from a more serious arterial disease called atherosclerosis.

This is a disease of the arterial wall in which deposits of fibrous and fatty substances, especially one called cholesterol, develop in the inner or lining layer of the arteries. These deposits narrow the channel and may even obstruct it entirely and present roughened surfaces on which blood clots can form and add their own form of arterial blockage.

Let's pause here a moment and consider the nature of cholesterol. It has become something of a dirty word in the vocabulary of the new fitness cults but cholesterol does not exist in your system with the sole object of killing you.

The association of blood fats, or plasma lipids, with atheroma and heart disease has been the subject of concentrated research which has considerably broadened knowledge and understanding of the human condition.

There are four forms of lipid in plasma: Saturated or unsaturated fatty acids; triglycerides, which make up 95 per cent of the lipids of adipose or fatty tissue; phospholids, complex lipids which contain phosphate and a nitrogenous base; and cholesterol, which occurs in two forms, high density and low density, and also comes from two sources — your intestine and by synthesis in your body.

Absorption from the intestine is roughly proportional to intake in the range found in the usual diet. In affluent societies, this is about 600 to 800 mg a day, mainly from meat, dairy products and particularly egg yolk. One egg contains about 250 mg of cholesterol. So there is no avoiding it. To a certain extent, high diet intakes of cholesterol are compensated by reduced synthesis.

The nature of the fat in your diet influences your cholesterol level. Saturated fatty acids, found chiefly in animal fats, as is cholesterol, increase plasma levels; polyunsaturated fatty acids, as in vegetable oils, tend to lower them.

But, at all ages and different levels, cholesterol exists; highest in affluent societies and highest, in those societies, among people in their fifth and sixth decades.

Atherosclerosis is a common condition in most countries. It particularly affects the arteries supplying the heart, the brain and the lower limbs but its appearance in one artery does not mean it must be present in all. Its occurrence is very patchy and quite unpredictable; it is possible, and common, for atherosclerosis to be present in marked degree in one small vessel and negligible elsewhere.

It is important to remember, too, that atherosclerosis may progress very slowly or not at all. People can and do live for 10, 15 or more years after it appears — and live quite actively. The most important site for atherosclerosis is in the coronary arteries which supply the heart and it is the greatest single cause of chronic ill-health in the United States, Canada, New Zealand, Australia and several other countries. But much can be done to prevent it.

The coronary arteries encircle the heart like a crown and their fine branches interlace in an elaborate irrigation system. If one or more of the branches are narrowed by athero-sclerosis, doctors use the short-term coronary sclerosis to define the problem. If a branch becomes completely blocked, it is a coronary occlusion. Usually, the final blocking process is due to a blood clot forming on the narrowed arterial wall and the term coronary thrombosis is applied. These last two terms essentially mean the same thing.

A sudden and complete stoppage of blood flow through a branch of the coronary system sometimes, but not always, causes part of the heart muscle, which gets its blood supply from that vessel, to weaken. The injured area is called a myocardial infarction; generally, it is a small area and does not significantly reduce the total bulk of the heart muscle.

Sometimes, a more extensive area is damaged but nature provides for the repair and replacement of these injuries just as it does in other tissues of the body. It forms a firm, fibrous scar exactly like the scar which heals a clean cut in the skin. As a rule, this scar causes no symptoms. Many people have them and never know; nor does the scar usually interfere with the function of the remaining heart muscle.

Some patients with a restriction in the coronary circulation develop a characteristic type of chest pain when they exert themselves beyond a certain limit. This pain stops quickly if they stand still. It is known as angina pectoris and it is important to distinguish this short-lived type of attack from the much longer pain which occurs in a coronary occlusion. Attacks of angina pectoris do not damage the heart. Patients who do not understand this believe each attack of pain provoked by effort signals a fresh heart attack.

This is quite wrong. Sir Thomas Lewis, one of the leading scientists in heart research, suffered from angina pectoris for 20 years and he is only one of many who have lived long and usefully despite the presence of a form of coronary disease.

So far, the basic cause of coronary disease remains unknown but many clues have been uncovered and, surprisingly, the fact that the frequency of the disease in countries such as ours has increased greatly in the past 50 years encourages doctors to believe they will ultimately find the cause and, from there, the prevention.

Half a century ago, most doctors regarded heart disease as part of the natural process of ageing and something they were powerless to stop or impede. When it became apparent that the disease occurred more frequently in some countries than it did in others, they argued that this was mainly due to better methods of diagnosis in those areas, especially through the discovery of the electro-cardiogram. Another argument was that generally longevity in those countries had been increased by the elimination of such killers as diphtheria, typhoid, tuberculosis and the complications of accidents, childbirth and surgery, by improved nutrition and living conditions. All this enabled people to live on into the age when coronary disease could be expected to appear. This may well explain some of the increase but, emphatically, not all of it.

One fairly well-established factor is a circumstance which affects the life pattern of the mass of the world's people — war. German doctors recorded that arterial disease seemed less at the end of World War One and in the few years of severe food shortage that followed. After World War Two, Norwegian doctors noted that heart disease began rising and linked this with a pre-war increase and a wartime decrease to point the finger at excess food consumption and lack of exercise — conditions which the war and the occupation years reversed.

It could well be that findings such as these will lead to

accurate diagnosis of just how our way of life is responsible for coronary disease and other diseases of the heart and arteries.

But we don't have to wait for the miracles. We can do things for ourselves as individuals. Like ridding our minds of some of the lay misconceptions and fallacies that obstruct many attitudes to the use and care of the heart and, as we read on, by putting on our jogging shoes.

The belief that a coronary means the end of useful, active life is widespread, even today — and wrong. Most coronary occlusions affect only a small branch of the coronary tree and the blocked vessel may be bypassed by collateral channels which lie unused in the tissues awaiting just this emergency. These can be so efficient that, after recovery, the patient may have no disability at all or else only on extreme exertion.

Must the patient with coronary disease rest all the time? No. In the acute phase of an attack, the healing process is helped if the body is rested; but, once healing is complete, further rest rarely achieves anything of value and is likely only to increase disability by adding the effects of physical unfitness and lack of self-confidence.

Is exertion harmful after a coronary attack? This is a variation of the same theme as the need for rest; it is usually just as wrong. The heart has enormous reserves of power which are not often used in ordinary living but enable people to perform prodigious feats — or to run a mile in less than four minutes and a marathon in less than 135 minutes.

After many coronary attacks, the reserve power is un-diminished and available for use. There will be symptoms of over-exertion — a special type of chest pain and breathless-ness — which are nature's way of signalling it is time to slow down but similar symptoms can be produced by physical unfitness or anxiety. The failure to distinguish between the two leads many patients to restrict their activities far too much.

3. Meet your enemies

N OW THAT YOU'VE been introduced to your best friend —
your heart — meet some of your worst enemies:
Overweight, underwork, cholesterol, atheroma and stress.

Overweight and underwork do not need any description,
just some realistic thought. They are two conditions we have
grown into through carelessness, through taking in far more
calories than our energy outputs require, through indulging
ourselves in far too many fatty foods, through inherited bad
eating habits.

Cholesterol and atheroma are two things that could stop
you in your tracks before you are old enough to die.
Atheroma is a degenerative change in the inner and middle
coats of the arteries, a condition of thickening and rigidity
which is a natural change in old age but which our way of life
can bring on prematurely.

Atheroma leads to partial blockage of the arteries and
restriction of the blood supply; to clotting, coronary thrombosis or apoplexy. As a next step, plates of lime may form in
the arteries or the arteries may deteriorate into brittle cal-
careous tubes very liable to tearing from the slightest injury.

Cholesterol is a substance derived from the many tissues of
the body — fat, blood, tumours and secretions such as bile.
In recent years, evidence has increased of a correlation
between a high level of cholesterol in the blood and coronary
heart disease.

These are two degenerative results of modern-day living —
stress has added an important and often unappreciated third.

You can be a good runner and eat all the right kinds of foods but still suffer from stress and end up having a heart attack. Under stress, you increase the blood sugars and cholesterol in the blood and this leads to high blood pressure.

The fact that modern living can and does lead to cardio-respiratory deterioration was brought home to me many years ago at an executive health conference in Australia, organised by the Australian Medical Assocation's industrial medicine division, which handed out the basic message that a gloomy prospect of heart disease plagues the life of all soft-living executives.

One speaker, Mr Alan J. Goble, honorary cardiologist of the Royal Melbourne Hospital, said: 'Countries proud of their high standard of living, such as the United States, Canada, the United Kingdom, Australia and New Zealand, have the highest incidence of heart disease. The lowest incidences are found in Africa and other under-developed countries. White South Africans have one of the highest rates in the world while among the native Bantu the condition is almost unknown.

'Repeated surveys in Britain confirm that the incidence of the disease is twice as great in the upper social and occupational groups as in the lower or heavy labouring groups.

'The man with a combination of overweight, high cholesterol and hypertension is almost certain to develop coronary heart disease if he does not have a stroke first. Life assurance figures are clear. It pays to be lean.

'A high saturated fat diet is the most important cause of coronary artery disease, disablement and death in this (Australian) community so far discovered.

'The average middle-aged Australian is a paunchy, soft individual, probably beery, who exercises by shouting abuse on Saturday afternoons.

'The naked eye examination of the hearts of United States soldiers killed in the Korean war disclosed coronary artery disease in two-thirds and occlusive atheroma in one-third. Yet the average age of the men was 22 years.

'Atheroma is not a part of the ageing process but a disease

21

related to a high standard of living in an advanced technical society. It is the most important single structural abnormality in the lives of most of us.

'In classic Greece, a man was expected to be fit for military service at 60 years. Agesilaus, King of Sparta, was still campaigning hard in the field, not merely directing battles, at the age of 80.'

Dr D. R. Wilson, chief medical officer for the Vacuum Oil Corporation, said: 'I've found that in every 100 persons over 40 who haven't taken a comprehensive medical test in the previous five years, at least 20 persons will have a significant medical condition of which they're unaware.

'This condition could affect health at the time, and the work performance, would certainly affect health in the future and might even shorten the life span.

'Many diseases which are discovered at the age of 40 begin much earlier. In coronary heart disease, the heart attack typically occurs about the age of 50 yet its origin could be traced back 5, 10 or 15 years.

'A man can be physically fit but in poor health. He may be tired, anxious, mildly depressed, in a rut, lacking in sleep, bored. Health is positive and there will be a sense of well-being. If a person is not healthy, then obviously he will be inefficient, unable to do his work properly and perhaps suffer from minor complaints of a non-physical origin.'

Dr Bryan J. Gandevia, senior fellow in industrial medicine at Melbourne University, said: 'Judicious exercise would improve the efficiency of lungs and heart at any age — but one round of golf or one game of squash or tennis a week is not a satisfactory training programme.'

A doctor once remarked to me that a blood test of the average citizen of western countries would show a far greater cholesterol condition than in the average citizen of countries generally labelled as undemocratic. Without being political, that is a staggering argument against democracy — or should I call it complacency.

We suffer from the deterioration of over-civilisation so seriously that immediate national health campaigns are of the utmost importance. East Germany woke up to this fact many years ago and established its national 'Run For Your Life' programme, which doubled the membership of all types of sports clubs and brought home to virtually every citizen the realisation that continued well-being rested in their hands and demanded positive action.

From this realisation and a vigorous approach to the study of sports medicine has grown the sensational emergence of the East Germans as an athletic force in recent Olympic and international contests.

Are they really that much better than we are? Or have they just got rid of complacency?

The western world's average person is accustomed to dropping interest in competitive sports and even in exercise in their early thirties, apart from spasmodic rounds of golf or games of squash and tennis. They move from the field of activity into the bleachers and watch others making the effort, reserving the right to sneer: They aren't as good as we were in our day.

What people overlook is that neither are they as good as they were in their day, and they are getting progressively worse. Unless they get off the seat of their pants and do something about it, they are heart disease candidates ahead of their time.

Fortunately, the widespread acceptance of jogging has dramatically altered that state of mind in the last decade or so because there has been a remarkable accompanying flow-on effect of the fitness it induced in veteran sporting activities which were unheard of in the 1960s and even the early 1970s.

Simply, to continue enjoying life, we have to keep our bodies in a reasonable condition and we can do it easily, by taking exercise a little at a time and often. If you operate a machine, you take constant care of it to keep it efficient. Think of your body as a machine and stop expecting it to go on ticking along without any attention and not even miss a beat at some of the abuses and neglect you show it.

Incidentally, on the subject of fat, there is one form, commonly known as brown fat, which is a positive asset. It is usually found in areas of the back and has the peculiar characteristic that, even while you are sleeping, it goes on burning up calories.

It makes you a warm-bodied person, it keeps your weight down without the need for dieting or other emergency measures, it enables you to eat pretty much what you like and in the quantities you choose without worrying about piling on excess weight.

If you're a brown fat person, you're lucky. If you are not, you are unlucky, because you can't go out and buy any.

4. The biggest killer is your heart

T HIS BOOK IS concerned primarily with the facts of life. And this involves also consideration of the facts of death.

Civilised countries go to endless expense, in time and money and ingenuity, to conduct the most creditable campaigns against the death and injury toll on the roads and in the water. Warnings, exhortations and publicity about the dangers of cancer, particularly of the lungs, are constant.

Not nearly as much attention is paid to the danger of heart troubles caused by poor living, bad eating and lack of exercise. More, perhaps, now that more people are becoming conscious of themselves physically and physiologically but we are talking about the problem that still removes most of us from this earth.

In 1961, accidents in New Zealand killed 4.39 people in every 10,000. Cancer killed 15.10. These were figures to justify campaigns, sure enough, but heart disease killed 31.98. In 1975, the comparative figures were 5.40, 16.45 and 26.81. The gap had narrowed but the disparity is still shockingly obvious.

Official New Zealand figures show that the 1961 death rate from heart disease was 186.5 per cent higher than it was in the 1900-09 period and 37.1 per cent higher than it was as recently as the decade before World War Two. Since 1968, there has been a steady decline in the death rate, of about 8 per cent on the figures for 1950-52 but it is still a safe bet that one in every four New Zealanders will die of heart disease.

As yet, there is no proof that the conversion of thousands

to jogging has anything to do with the decline but it would be nice to think so and, perhaps, it will be proved one day to have played a significant part.

Meantime, it remains an appalling thought that in New Zealand, long regarded as one of the most favoured countries in the world, about five people drop dead from heart disease for every one killed in a road accident. New Zealand has one of the world's highest road vehicle counts in proportion to population but it is not the volume of traffic we have to fear most as our killer. Nor is cancer.

The American scene is no prettier. In 1973, cancer killed 351,924 Americans. Accidents killed 116,297, pneumonia and influenza 65,599, diabetes 38,225 and other causes 342,428. Diseases of the heart and blood vessels killed 1,062,160. About 260,000 of heart deaths were of people under 65 — American statistics match those of New Zealand and other countries in showing that heart disease is striking earlier and earlier in people's lives.

In that year, 1973, cardio-vascular disease was calculated to have cost the United States $22.7 billion; a total of 28,830,000 Americans were estimated to have some form of heart and blood vessel disease; and one in six suffered from hypertension.

Every year, some 350,000 Americans die of heart attacks before they reach hospital. Some 23 million have high blood pressure — but only 50 per cent are aware of it. The cardio-vascular disease rate is 481.3 in 100,000. The equivalent New Zealand rate is about 300 and we think that is shockingly high.

Unpalatable facts about how we treat — or ill-treat — ourselves are not in short supply. In 1972, a survey in the New Zealand community of Napier of people between 21 and 92 showed 20 per cent had suffered or were suffering from hypertension. In the even smaller town of Milton, 31 per cent of the men and 50 per cent of the women in the 60-69 age group had raised blood pressure.

These surveys post the warnings but they are often ignored. In another survey in New Zealand, for example, 121 people were advised to see their doctors, but only 89 bothered. Even the routine and entirely comfortable process of having one's blood pressure checked seems to be too much trouble.

Many comparative studies of occupational effects on the heart have been made. Bus drivers have been compared with conductors, post office clerks with postmen, office workers with factory floor workers. Every study has produced the same answer: A pattern of lower incidence of and mortality from coronary heart disease among the more active groups.

Of particular importance was a 1977 report which followed a 22-year study of the occurrence of fatal heart attacks among 3686 San Francisco longshoremen. It showed that those in sedentary jobs ran an 80 per cent greater risk of fatal heart attack than those who lifted, shoved and stacked all the time. The active ones exhausted about 1800 calories a day above the basic rate.

When the study began in 1951, some 60 per cent of the longshoremen were in the hard work group. By 1972, because of the introduction of forklifts, containers, push-button cranes, conveyers and other mechanical aids, only 5 per cent remained in the hard work group.

The study concluded that low work output was just as influential in increasing the risk of a fatal coronary heart disease as cigarette smoking and high blood pressure and much more influential than obesity, diabetes or high cholesterol. During the 22 years, the hard work group recorded 18.2 per cent fatal heart attacks. The low energy sedentary group, which was growing steadily in number, had a 41.2 per cent record.

So, if we sit down to work, what can we do about it? Yet another study established that civil servants who travelled by car from door to door each working day were twice as likely to show indications of pending heart trouble in electro-cardiograms as men in the same occupational group who walked for 20 minutes or more.

Up to the middle of last century, the general belief existed that exercise was a potential cause of cardiac damage. Incredibly, this belief still has a few strongholds.

Sports medicine researchers Ernst and Peter Jokl, of the

University of Kentucky and Yale University Medical Schools, wrote in 1977 that, as late as 1901, leading English doctors were combining to condemn all runs of more than one mile by high school boys. Girls were not mentioned because it was thought that they should not run at all. This kind of warning was never substantiated but the man in the street listened and reacted by inaction. To some extent, they still do so today.

In 1935, F. W. Lempriere analysed the medical records of 16,000 schoolboys covering a period of 30 years. This impressive study led to the conclusion, which startled the medical profession, that heart strain through exercise is practically unknown. Lempriere mentioned six fatalities in 20 years; four were due to accidents, one was a football player who died two hours after a meal and the other was a boy who high-jumped eight days after an attack of tonsilitis and died seven months later from infective endocarditis.

Coming on top of a flood of 'authoritative' papers in school health and physical education publications warning of 'heart strain through exercise', this was a devastating contradiction but, say Jokl and Jokl, 'in the light of the facts as we now know them, the papers read like Hans Christian Andersen's fairy tale of the emperor's invisible clothes. No clinical information and autopsy protocols were presented to support the allegations that heart disease can be caused by exercise. In fact, we now know that the hearts of young athletes are singularly capable to adjust themselves to strenuous exercise. This statement applies to children in general and to girls in particular.

'It is of exceptional relevance,' they continue, 'for the evaluation of athletic feats such as that of a 15-year-old East German girl, Petra Thumer, who in 1976 at Montreal established a new world record for swimming 400m freestyle in 4:09.89, thus equalling the winning time in the men's event at the Tokyo Olympic Games in 1964. There can be no doubt that the medical prophets of doom possessed more eloquence than knowledge.'

It is of considerable significance to the approach to jogging for everyone that, in recent years, with the discovery that women can absorb training loads as demanding as those formerly considered suitable only for mature men, women's times in running and swimming events calling for both speed and endurance have been lowered far more dramatically than the comparative times for men. Consider, for instance, that in the past two years, women have reduced their best marathon times from over 2:40 to less than 2:30 and are now within 15 minutes of matching the best men at the distance.

The women athletes of East Germany were a classic example of the ability of women to respond to training. Another was provided in 1978 when a Danish girl, Loa Olafsson, carved 58 seconds from the world 10,000 metres record of Rumania's Natalia Marasescu. Loa was then only 20, had been training under my direction for only two years and was already Denmark's 800, 1500 and 3000 metres champion.

Quoting Jokl and Jokl again: 'A major contribution of clinical sports medicine in cardiology has been the clarification of the categorical distinction between the ageing process as against the natural history of diseases which occur with conspicuous frequency in older people. Chief among the latter is coronary atherosclerosis causing myocardial degeneration. Physical training modifies all facets of the ageing process. It decelerates the decline of physique, the decline of fitness and — within strict limits — the decline of health, such as the rate of progress of the ischemic heart diseases.'

Jokl and Jokl point out that a number of athletes over 40 have reached Olympic finals. Several grandmothers have won Olympic medals. In the Honolulu marathon of 1974, a 67-year-old university professor won the senior class contest, covering the 42 kilometres in just under four hours. He began preparation for the race only after his 64th birthday, before which he had led a sedentary life. Three years of conscientiously pursued daily training enabled him to perform this extraordinary feat of endurance. The 1975 Boston marathon was contested by a group of middle-aged men who a few years earlier had been afflicted with myocardial infarction. All of them were trained at the Toronto Rehabilitation Centre.

Jokl and Jokl say: 'The quality of the lives of physically fit

29

elderly persons is certainly superior to that of men and women who spend their declining years in homes for the aged. It must be added in this context that the decision of "senior citizens" as to whether to participate in running and other physical activities is not necessarily made on medical grounds alone.

'In 1967, we attended a medical congress on physical activity and ageing held in Israel ... We had the opportunity to watch a "three-day march to Jerusalem", an annual contest in which every participant must walk 25 kilometres a day. Among the 40,000 entries was a man 100 years of age.

'He completed the course. We congratulated him after the event and asked: "Was it not a remarkable decision for a man of your age to enter this contest?" To this, he replied: "What better death could I hope for than to die on the way to Jerusalem?" '

It would be possible to continue quoting evidence for several more chapters but we think that, if you have read this far, you should need no more convincing. It is time now to stop absorbing the reasons why you should begin thinking of yourself as a jogger and begin the active process of becoming one. It is not much more difficult than sitting back reading this book — but only you can make the decision to tackle that degree of difficulty.

5. Fatness, fitness and fatigue

D IET, PHYSICAL ACTIVITY and emotional stress are factors which must be considered in discussing heart disease. We'll consider them one by one for their relative importance.

The complete answer on the role of diet in coronary disease is not known but, generally speaking, in countries where the diet is, theoretically, poor and lacking in animal products — Africa and Asia, for example — the incidence of coronary disease is lower than in prosperous countries where a full variety of food is available. Also, the richer members of communities that are generally poor are more affected by coronary disease than their poorer compatriots.

The argument that the apparent low rate in those countries was due to natural or racial immunity was upset long ago by the discovery that American Negroes, especially those living in big cities, suffer a high rate of coronary disease. Years ago, too, it was discovered that the rate among Japanese in Hawaii was far higher than in their relatives at home. It was higher still among prosperous Japanese living in California. And, since Japan's postwar economic boom has vaulted its living standards upwards, medical authorities have reported a rising rate of coronary disease there.

Another argument against the diet theory is that in poor countries the death rate from other diseases, particularly those related to malnutrition and infection, is high so that a smaller percentage of the populative survives to the age when coronary disease becomes prevalent.

This was countered by a study of special populations —

the Trappist and Benedictine monks. The Trappists lead a most austere life and follow a vegetarian diet; the Benedictine monks indulge in a richer diet. The Benedictines were found to have a much higher rate of coronary disease than the Trappists.

For years, it has been known that coronary disease is much more common in people who are overweight. This all suggests that diet is an important factor but, because our total health is so dependent on what and how we eat, we have to be careful of making drastic diet alterations.

Evidence is growing, based on overseas investigations, that the great increase in coronary disease in this country is due, at least in part, to the damaging effects of emotional stress which arise from our sophisticated and technologically fast-moving way of life. It had been accepted until recently that the degree of stress would have to become almost unbearable before it would become dangerous, but it seems evident now that a way of life in which continual anxiety and stress are present does lead to all the symptoms of heart disease. You can, in fact, worry yourself into an early grave.

We can be a lot more positive about the role of physical inactivity in coronary disease. It could well be a major factor behind the booming heart failure statistics in prosperous industrialised countries — an idea which may surprise those many people who still attribute a heart attack to a lifetime of hard work or some excessive physical strain.

Evidence is strong that coronary disease in any community is highest among those whose life is sedentary, and lowest among those whose occupation involves strenuous work. In some countries, and the United States is a classic example, mechanisation has advanced so far and the physical effort involved in occupation, travel, housework and leisure has been reduced so much that few people, young or old, lead a life of adequate activity.

In short, the prevalence of coronary disease runs parallel with the mechanisation of work, transport and leisure — our technological experts, for instance, have made it no longer necessary to even get up to switch television channels. Add the additional factors of over-eating, stress, excessive consumption of alcohol and tobacco and we have a powerful mutual conspiracy to rob us of our greatest asset, physical fitness.

So what can we do to protect ourselves?

As we've said, it is potentially dangerous to alter habitual diet drastically except on a doctor's advice, particularly for anyone with already established coronary disease. Every patient presents special problems only his doctor can know or understand.

But certain principles of diet can be followed and none of us is too old or too young to adopt them and to benefit from them. The rules apply with special force to anyone who has or suspects heart disease, has good reason to believe they are prone to arterial disease, or is overweight.

The food we eat provides the chemicals from which muscle, bone, blood tissue and all other tissues are built. The main groups we need are proteins, fats, carbohydrates, minerals and enzymes. We also need a large number of additives — chemicals used in tiny amounts to assist our chemical processes to run smoothly. These are the vitamins which are easily destroyed by modern food-processing methods and by many of our cooking habits. Enzymes, too, are at risk; some can withstand heat but some cannot; some come from the body itself; some we manufacture and some come from the natural foods we eat.

For most people, the essential foodstuffs would be provided each day by about four to eight ounces (100 to 200 grams) of lean meat, one or two ounces (25 to 50 grams) of cheese, an egg, half a pint (300 ml) of milk, some fresh fruit and green vegetables. Is that all you eat?

Additional calories, mainly provided by carbohydrates, will vary with energy output, age, sex, constitution, body build and occupation. You can settle your personal doubts by talking them over with your doctor and you can also profitably read a little on the subject, providing you don't get hooked on books written by food faddists, cranks and extremists.

Over-eating is probably the biggest health problem for most people in the western world, except for that cross-section of the elderly and lonely who, from apathy and depression, eat less and less, choose food which needs little or no preparation, because it is easier, and expose themselves to malnutrition.

Obviously, the food needs of a growing child, a young woman rearing children and a man doing heavy manual work are quite different from those of adults in sedentary jobs. Yet, very often, the food habits we build early in life never change; we don't bother or see the need to change them. When, as life becomes easier, we should be eating less, we are often, because the helpings get bigger, eating more.

Large meals impose considerable strain on the digestion, cause the level of fatty substances in the blood stream to rise excessively and demand from the heart the same sort of performance as strenuous exertion to supply large volumes of blood to the digestive system. Yet, more and more, our lifestyle encourages hurried, skimpy feeding during the day and concentration on a veritable orgy of eating at night.

Many housewives still make the preparation of a large meal their greatest interest because they feel it is how best they can show their devotion. It is killing by kindness, particularly if the man of the house is an executive in the habit of indulging in executive lunches.

Take a lesson and a warning from the birds. They eat little and often, and scientists have found that they rarely suffer from arterial disease unless they are kept in captivity. Then, like us, they face two of the evils of modern life — overfeeding and inactivity.

We should eat slowly and make meal-time a part of leisure activity. Doctors who have studied what happens to sugar and fatty substances after a meal is digested know that small meals eaten in a relaxed way satisfy the appetite more than large quantities of food manfully forced down.

Appetite — or inherent greed — tends to diminish because, as small meals become a habit, the wide swings in the blood's sugar level — which promote appetite — are overcome. The level of fatty substance in the blood is also kept to a minimum.

Can you imagine an athlete eating a hearty meal before

entering a contest? And why don't they? Because the increased work the digestion of that meal would demand from the heart would seriously affect performance. Apply that thinking to your own way of life.

The average middle-aged American is about 20 lbs (9 kg) above ideal weight. The New Zealand counterpart was, a few years ago, rapidly overhauling that figure. Far too many still are, but many thousands have been converted. Overweight is a serious medical problem because it increases the risk of several serious diseases, including coronary disease, high blood pressure and diabetes. For the patient with established heart disease, the problem is even more urgent.

Consider this — a person 28 lbs (13 kg) overweight is loading the heart, muscle and joints with the equivalent of half a sack of potatoes. Try carrying that on your back all day.

Your best weight is what we could call your fighting weight — your lowest weight when you were young and fit. That is where you should aim to stay right through life. Gaining weight with age is not natural or inevitable. It is essentially due to a food intake in excess of energy output. We get older, we exert ourselves less and operate at a lower overall tempo; therefore, less energy is consumed but our appetite for food, built up over a lifetime, does not normally decrease in proportion. Often, it increases because we have more time for nibbling and we indulge in food sometimes as a compensation for failing powers in other directions.

So, if we want to avoid trouble in later life, we should tackle the problem early in life by a strong determination to avoid weight gain with age. We need an understanding of the problem as well as determination because, without understanding, attempts at weight reduction are rarely successful except for short periods.

We must get weight off and keep it off. It is not easy but it is governed by three basic rules:
1. Do more.
2. Eat less.
3. Weigh daily.

Doctors today put more emphasis on rule 1. because studies have shown that overweight people tend to reduce energy output in proportion to their excess of poundage. This was proved when a group of children was secretly filmed playing a ball game in a school-yard. The film showed that the lean children chased the ball enthusiastically but the overweight ones simply waited for it to come within reach. This was not a case of simple laziness but revealed a difference in temperament and outlook which could constitute a lifelong problem.

It can lead us, for example, to choose an occupation requiring little energy output. In London, many years ago, tests on bus drivers and conductors showed that coronary trouble was twice as prevalent among the drivers. The conductors were on their feet and active; the drivers were sitting down.

But the interesting discovery of the study was that, even on entry into the transport company's service, the drivers tended to be fatter than the conductors. They preferred the sit-down role, which indicated they were pandering to their condition and giving themselves a useful start along the road to serious heart problems.

If you are young and overweight and the job you do is sedentary, you have to make the conscious effort to take exercise, to move as much as possible, to learn to do things the hard active way.

Because reduced food intake is also necessary for reduced weight, you should acquire a reasonable knowledge and understanding of the simple principles of nutrition, otherwise you may deprive your body ultimately of essential foodstuffs needed for healthy functioning. You should not have any more difficulty in learning about the inner workings of your body than about the innards of your automobile — and which knowledge, in the long run, is more valuable? You CAN buy a new car.

It helps to know the energy value of the common foodstuffs. This is calculated in units called calories and the number of calories in an item of food is the amount of energy that food will provide after digestion.

If the total calorie intake exceeds the energy output, the surplus will be stored as fat. The average person in a sedentary job needs about 2000 calories a day; a man doing heavy manual work may need up to 4000. An excess of about 600 calories a day beyond energy output can add about a pound (400 grams) of fat.

No-one with heart disease should try to reduce weight suddenly and drastically. A slow, sure campaign is safer for everyone; but, of course, it is more difficult.

Drugs which suppress appetite or increase metabolism to burn off excess calories are rarely safe if used for long periods. And their effect is short-lived.

An indispensable item in every reducing campaign is the bathroom scale. Get on it every day — but get on it naked. You cannot fool yourself in the face of the bare truth it reveals. You cannot exaggerate the weight of your clothing or the small change in your pocket as justification for that extra weight you know you shouldn't have.

It is even more important to weigh daily once you've got your weight back to the desired level. As soon as an increase of 2 lb appears, cut down food severely until the ideal weight is restored.

You are physically fit when your body is capable of performing near to its limit of endurance without distress. Physical fitness not only protects us from many illnesses, it increases the feeling of well-being we call good health and condition and on which our efficiency and happiness largely depends.

Sadly, physical fitness is the exception rather than the rule in people after middle life. This is a problem of national importance in many countries; let us not shirk that point. Unfitness saps our health, our morale and our chances of ultimate survival as a nation.

It need not. Physical fitness can be regained easily by training, which means regular and repeated performance of exercise. In general, this exercise must tax your physical endurance to some degree. Young people won't get fit playing croquet or bowls; they have got to put a greater demand on the heart, lungs and muscles. As we age, we can be less strenuous, but that need remains to push ourselves physically, every day if possible.

There is one simple, economical, enjoyable way in which we choose our own time, our own place and our own pace. By jogging.

6. Where jogging was born

I F YOU'RE WONDERING why we hold such strong views on the value of jogging, you have only to look about you these days and see the people who are jogging and getting benefit from it. Talk to them if you can; ask them what they feel now that they didn't feel before they began.

Most likely, one way or another, they will echo the thoughts and convictions that led me to preach jogging for health more than two decades ago, when I was a bit of a voice in the wilderness whenever the subject of endurance or stamina training came up. What was the basis of my knowledge or for my contentions and opinions in those days? Simply, that I knew myself. I was an addict from long experience and I was eager to see my addiction infect others.

I gained my raw understanding of the physical limits and benefits of exercise at first hand, in the process of combating my own unfitness and then of adapting my personal training habits for the benefit of athletes who were attracted to train with me. It began 37 years ago, when I was 27, a winter footballer and a summer swimmer-cum-athlete who, like most New Zealanders, didn't train with any diligence or purpose because I believed I was fit through taking part in competition.

But then, a friend who was an experienced distance runner, talked me into a six-mile run and showed me how far from real fitness I was. My pulse rate rose rapidly. I blew hard and gasped for air. My lungs and throat felt as if they'd been scorched. My legs were like rubber. My whole body felt the effects of the run and of the effort expended in getting me to the end of it.

Thousands who have since turned to jogging to regain youthful fitness will identify easily with those reactions. They, too, will have run too fast and too far for their condition, as I admit I did, because they didn't appreciate how unfit — in the true sense of the word — they had become.

I could puff and pant through the stop-start of a football game, but I learnt that sustained running threw a strain on my body that seasons of football had not prepared me for.

I could have gone through the agony of recovery and then forgotten the experience but, instead, I began thinking about the cause of it and came to the question: If I'm reduced to this state by that run at 27, what will I be like at 47?

Possibly, that moment of truth was the birth-point of jogging because I then began a routine of daily running, curious to find out how it would affect me and how it would benefit me most in the long term. I had drawn the logical conclusion from the six-miler that sustained running, if tackled with less impetuosity and more preparation, would benefit my general health by working markedly on my respiratory and blood circulation systems; but I wanted to know how and why.

Within a few months of fairly controlled running, I was comfortably covering up to 15 miles (24 kilometres); but, being a dogmatic, stubborn and, I suppose, thorough person, I still wasn't satisfied that I was going about it the right way. So I began running to extremes, seeing how far I could run and what pressures of pace my body could stand. I discovered my physical limits by exceeding them.

The process went on for many years while I became an active and fairly successful middle and distance runner and, from it all, evolved my marathon-type endurance training system which is now internationally accepted as one of the most significant stepping-stones to greater athletic achievement. Out of it grew a new understanding of human physiology in relation to athletic endeavour; and from that flowed a new race of world champions, for several years led by the few athletes who first joined me on training runs.

From it, too, evolved the principles of jogging.

I got there the hard way; now it is simple. I have reduced it to a basic and understandable formula. The theories I tested and proved on myself and my early runners like Peter Snell, Murray Halberg and company many years ago, have since been tested again and confirmed by physiologists and sports medicine experts all over the world. They are being put into practice every day by a growing number of middle and distance runners, by sportspeople in all fields of activity who want to add the extra quality of stamina to their skills, and by millions of people who are purely and simply fit and healthy joggers.

The individual records of Lydiard-system trained athletes are well known and constantly chronicled; they are not important to this book except as confirmation that the system works. It made me, five years after that awful six-mile run, the New Zealand marathon champion and Empire Games marathon representative.

It also enabled me, 34 years later and without specifically training for it, to run a 2:58.58 marathon at the age of 61.

7. Stamina ... not strength

S TAMINA IS THE whole and simple answer to the business of fitness. Stamina, not strength, produces the essential state of tirelessness which is the hallmark of the really fit person.

Strength involves lifting an exceptional weight once, twice or a given number of times; stamina involves lifting a lesser weight an indefinite number of times.

Ask the biggest muscle man in your community to run a mile as fast as he can and the chances are he will wind up on the ground exhausted with most of the mile still to run; unless he is a strongman who has learnt to run as an element of his training.

Stamina is the capacity for sustained work through a general conditioning of the cardio-respiratory system and a systematic toning up of the muscles generally — not a deliberate building up of the specific muscles in the body which govern the ability to lift weight.

You don't add strength to the runner to enable him to run a mile in less than four minutes. He almost certainly already has the speed; what stamina gives him is the ability to sustain that inherent speed for the required distance. Peter Snell was a fast runner before he became my pupil; I gave him the stamina to maintain that speed better and longer than others who were basically faster but could not sustain their pace.

The group of New Zealanders who met for the first organised jog in 1961 were all capable, or had been capable, of running at reasonable speeds. All of them had lost that capacity. Among their ample stomachs and double chins —

they averaged about 47 years of age — was so little true fitness that most of them could barely stagger a quarter of a mile. The years of inactivity and neglect hit them in the lungs and muscles like a sledgehammer.

Before they began their initial jog, I warned them against becoming too competitive and they laughed. None could visualise that such a thing could happen; and they could picture it even less a quarter of a mile later.

But after three months some of those joggers entered as a team in a relay race, involving each in one and a quarter laps of a racecourse, with hurdles, against young full-time athletes — and they were not the last to finish. Eight months later, seven of them finished a marathon.

One 240-pounder (110 kg) who began with a pulse rate of 80 fined down in eight months to 168 lbs (77 kg), with a 50 heart beat and the ability to run 26 miles (42 kilometres) or more without undue effort.

All of them proved that an agonised amble could quickly become a decent jogging speed. They became runners in the true sense of the word, discovering that it took only determined effort and patience, and that the rewards were freedom from illness, more energy for work and relaxation, release from physical and mental tiredness and a whole new outlook on life.

Their personal triumphs as joggers were exceptional stories in those days. They are commonplace now. Then, it was a rare sight to see a runner of more than 45 or 50 stepping out in a marathon race; today, it is usual for the veterans to outnumber the young runners in marathons all over the world. Many of them are women. There has to be a good reason for it all.

8. Your pulse is your health meter

J OGGERS GENERALLY HAVE been pleasantly surprised to notice dramatic reductions in their pulse rates over a period of steady sustained jogging. What is the significance of this? What happens inside the body when it is stimulated and exercised by jogging?

The pulse rate indicates, to a degree, the general condition of the body. Nature keeps everything balanced. So, if the heart is doing its job easily, so is every other vitally related organ in the body.

A high at-rest pulse rate generally means arteries are in a cholesterol condition or are under-developed, with a lack of elasticity. They could well be clogged with a deposit of fatty tissues on the lining, which restricts the flow of blood to various parts of the body and forces the heart to pump harder to push the required volume of blood past them.

Jogging speeds up the flow of blood and increases the pressure of the flow. This forced pressure at a higher temperature can cause a flushing action which can eradicate some fats and wastes from the arteries and out of the body. Exercise also uses the cholesterol as a source of energy when the energy is intense. Purdue University in Lafayette, Indiana, checked the cholesterol level of swimmers and then put them through a hard anaerobic workout. The cholesterol level of their blood was then found to be high; but some hours later it had returned to normal.

In distance runners, cholesterol is virtually non-existent when they are resting because of their continuous training

44

and the related continuous flushing of the system which prevents it from gaining a foothold by burning it up in the arterial system. The food intake may not be vastly different from anyone else's; it is just that what could be dangerous for the inactive person has no chance to establish itself in the active one.

As the cholesterol level is reduced, the flow of blood activated by exercise is given an easier passage, which allows the heart to throttle back. It stays throttled back when the body is relaxed between periods of exercise, so down comes the pulse rate. Its slowing is further helped because, as the arteries adjust to that frequent accelerated blood flow, they become more elastic and actually grow larger. The heart also tends to grow, retaining a proportion of the expansion caused by steady exercise.

Yet another factor is this: In the average person taking little exercise of a specialised nature and none at all of a general nature, the arterial system within those muscles which are not greatly used tends to be confined or restricted.

Running, because it affects most of the muscles of the body in one degree or another, causes an expansion of the arterial system. Veins and arteries which had ceased operation through inactivity and capillary networks which may never have operated at all are opened and put to constant use. With more channels for the blood to follow, easy blood flow becomes easier still.

And, if there should be any blockage in the system, the extended avenues for blood flow provide detours which considerably lessen the risk of harmful interruptions. It is this unhindered blood flow, pumped along by a heart ticking over comparatively gently, coupled with a toned-up muscular system and a conditioned cardio-respiratory system, that makes daily life so much easier.

It has been calculated that there can be 20 times the difference between the vascular system of the sedentary person and the one who does a good volume of aerobic exercise.

However, we must make the point that, irrespective of age or sex, we are all individuals and each of us has to be treated individually. Several people in their twenties have had strokes and died in fun runs through poor development of their cardiac systems. Possibly, unaware that they were at risk, they would have expended more energy and taken less heed of any warning signs than an older person, who would be wiser in the sense that he would expect or be on guard against indications that a younger person would ignore.

We give the warning now: Whatever your age, before you begin jogging, you must see your doctor, tell him what you want to do and ask him to check for any physical disability which would either prevent you from jogging safely or endanger you if you did jog.

Remember that as the muscles of the body operate on oxygen and blood, so does the brain. As the muscles become fitter, our reflexes become quicker, and our ability to think and act quickly and freshly is improved. We can do a better day's work because our mental and physical health enables us to keep going at a steady pitch without those tired backs, fogged minds and headaches that afflict so many workers around the middle of the afternoon.

Shock, stress or the sudden sprint for the after-work bus are dangerous to the unfit person because of a restricted cardio-respiratory system. The sudden stimulus causes a rapid surge in blood flow and pressure and, if the system isn't conditioned to take it, results in spots before the eyes, alarming palpitations and that feeling of faintness that sends the victim scurrying to a doctor seeking a cure for a weak heart. Or else the subject just drops dead immediately.

The person conditioned on a diet of distance jogging is cushioned by an elastic system against the upheaval of shock or sharp sprinting. They are also far more likely to catch that bus. The healthier heart and cardio-respiratory and vascular systems all lead to improved oxygen uptake — the ability of the system to assimilate oxygen, transport it and use it.

When the sprinter flings himself over 100 metres, blood pours through him at the rate of about 56 pints (32 litres) or more a minute, eight to ten times the flow the arterial system normally handles. Consider, therefore, how many hundreds of litres must circulate through someone running steadily for 20 miles (32 kilometres), or even for 15 minutes. Then you'll realise what a wonderful organ the heart is to be able to maintain this supply almost indefinitely. The pressure is tremendous — but all you have to do is keep your heart in a state of readiness for it.

It is designed to work many times harder than it does in normal conditions and it will do it cheerfully if you look after it and its related circulation system. Neglect it and your call for the several-times extra effort is going to be answered with total collapse or at least a pulse rate that pounds up in the hundreds and makes you feel as if your last days are approaching at a full gallop.

Almost certainly, whatever your personal oxygen uptake level is, it can be improved. Some doctors have claimed that the normal oxygen uptake of the individual cannot be improved beyond a certain level but I disagree. Most tests have been made on runners who have not been running for 20 or 30 years and the long-term physiological effects of running are not yet fully understood.

About 10 years ago I began training an American, Steve Goldberg, who told me then that he had never previously taken part in sporting activity. He was 38 and interested in jogging and asked if I would help him to get going. I trained him by correspondence for about two years and, at 40, he won the U.S. Masters' marathon in just over 2:32. He was a spectacular example of dedication to jogging and of physiological improvement.

New Zealander John Robinson was probably one of the slowest runners among the youngsters I have trained. He seemed to be devoid of natural talent but he loved to run and he has continued running ever since. He had been running for 20 years when, at 35, he won the New Zealand marathon title in 2:15. At 40, he won the world veterans' marathon title in West Germany in just over 2:20. So we have to be careful in making judgements about the general cardiac development of athletes over long terms. The limit would seem to have a certain infinity.

In well-trained athletes like Henry Rono, Sebastian Coe or John Walker, the oxygen uptake level would be seven litres or more a minute; the sedentary person could have a level of less than a litre. For them, walking up a few steps is an experience in breathlessness. But give that person a programme that requires maintaining aerobic exercise for 15 minutes or longer a day and, because of the pressure generally placed by the stimulated heart on the circulation and blood vascular systems, the ability to take in, transport and use oxygen leaps upward quite dramatically.

We tend to breathe a lot of oxygen in and straight out again because our systems are incapable of assimilating all of it. But if we develop our circulatory systems seven-fold or more — the difference between a Rono and an untrained person proves this is possible — and if we use certain muscle groups often for long periods, our use of oxygen and blood sugars and our elimination of wastes become most efficient. It would be difficult for anyone, even a cardiologist, to say positively what the limits are in any individual, of whatever age or sex, providing there are no restricting health problems, to exercise in this aerobic method.

When you're at rest, your arteries are in a contracted state. Therefore, the businessperson who walks only from their front door to the garage and from their car to the office desk and back again each day has arteries that are virtually in a contracted state all the time. No real pressure is being applied because they even avoid walking up a single flight of stairs if they can find an elevator. It is an escape from effort that is by no means confined to the middle-aged and elderly, either.

Like a balloon, the vascular system expands when pressure is forced into it. And, like a balloon, frequent expansion and contraction will eventually result in the system stretching until it is always bigger than its original collapsed state.

When you jog for, say, half an hour a day, most days of the week, the sustained pressure on the system adds elasticity, increases the normal contracted capacity, and, therefore, permits a greater and easier flow of blood at all times. A simple thing but a positive step towards shielding yourself from unwanted cholesterol and atheroma.

A heart specialist has told me he is convinced that a person who has lived a sedentary life and then jogs 30 minutes a day for 18 months could expect to double their general cardiac efficiency. Why don't you?

Let's examine another aspect of the body which is remarkably improved by jogging — the blood's red corpuscles. These are little things but there are plenty of them — between 5 and 6 million to the cubic millimetre and with a total surface area in the body of about three quarters of an acre, which is 15 times greater than the body's own surface area.

Their main job is to carry a substance called haemoglobin which combines in the blood with oxygen and, in this form, is the agent which oxidises the body's energy food, glycogen. Glycogen is stored in the liver and the muscles and, obviously, its efficiency depends on the capacity of the blood to carry to it the amount of oxygen required to oxidise it.

As long as the degree of muscular activity is moderate, the normal oxygen intake during respiration is sufficient but, when more strenuous exercise, like a fast three-mile (five-kilometre) run, is taken, the normal oxygen intake is not enough. Under these conditions, the glycogen doesn't oxidise but converts to lactic acid, a reaction which provides energy but doesn't need oxygen. This cannot go on for long because as the lactic acid accumulates it affects the muscles adversely, leading to fatigue and, ultimately, to a cessation of muscular contractions.

This is the state known as oxygen debt and it is a condition which slows up and exhausts the unfit person when they first take to running and, in fact, governs all athletic effort.

The point at which the oxygen debt begins to take over is called the maximum steady state and my distance-running programme is designed basically to lift that steady state progressively so that effort without oxygen debt can be maintained longer and steadily increased.

Another pair of words now familiar to most athletes are aerobic and anaerobic running. It is aerobic (with oxygen) and desirable for both distance-running training and jogging when you run beneath but as close as possible to your maximum steady state. It is anaerobic (without oxygen) when the running pace exceeds the maximum steady state and begins to create the oxygen debt.

Athletes have periods in their training when they are

obliged to go beyond their maximum steady state in effort and run anaerobically. Joggers should not — the secret of their aerobic running is that it systematically and without distress forces that maximum steady state to climb higher and higher and enable greater performance without noticeably greater effort.

The state of oxygen indebtedness must be deliberately avoided. No mad sprinting over the last 100 metres, for instance. No racing your jogging friends either to see who is fittest.

I reached my maximum steady state conclusions long before I became involved with sports medicine experts and physiologists who could help me. I've since become involved in the physiology of running myself through sharing my practical experience with their theory.

Most of us are fine as long as we are young and burning up our energy. But when we stop that energy consumption, we go on taking the energy-producing foods and cluttering ourselves up with the excesses. As long as we do that, we can expect atheroma, cholesterol, overworked hearts and all the other troubles that follow, in logical sequence, the build-up of fatty deposits in our systems.

Too many of us, as we grow older, make the mistake of coddling our hearts. We avoid doing strenuous things because we fear we might strain ourselves. We forget what we accepted without thought in our youth — that the body has the capacity to work under considerably more pressure than most of us give it credit for or are willing to apply to it.

How else can a 65-year-old, on a diet of aerobic running, suddenly canter through a full marathon when, five years earlier, he or she wouldn't dream of running a quarter-mile down the road and, probably, would avoid even walking it? He or she has got the same heart, the same body; just taken in hand and on foot and conditioned back to some of its lost youthfulness.

A doctor once told me: 'Everyone at some time in life has a blocked artery.' He'd extensively studied the muscles of dead people and found that the muscular systems of ex-athletes and physically active people showed evidence of blockage in some areas; but he also found a much more complex system of arteries and veins than sedentary workers had, which enabled them to bypass problem areas without even knowing they existed.

This doctor also concluded that jogging as an investment had a long-term benefit. Even if it was abandoned after a period, its benefit would last almost indefinitely with only slight and slow regression. This was a conclusion I had also reached. Both the ex-athlete and the sedentary worker might experience blood clots but the active person had far more chance of avoiding trouble.

This is a brief and simplified explanation of what happens to our bodies when we exercise and when we don't. The reactions described are quite apart from the other gains — the stretching, loosening, suppling and strengthening of our muscles, the development of better muscle fibre, and a beneficial reaction on all other bodily functions. They are all worthwhile but, for people who want to stay fit as they grow old, efficient internal systems are far more important than all the muscles in the world.

Those people who want to be healthy don't need a great mass of muscle. What they need are sound respiratory and blood systems. To get them and not the other, they must evaluate exercise carefully and choose those forms which direct their greatest benefit to the building of the important systems.

Remember, too, that the blood vascular and respiratory systems have a close mutual association, uniting in the common purpose of supplying oxygen to the tissues and removing carbon dioxide.

Jogging works directly on those systems, lifting the haemoglobin content of the blood, improving blood tone, enabling better oxygen absorption, transport and use, enlarging and expanding the arterial system, increasing the heart's capacity and reducing the demands on it at the same time, flushing out unwanted and dangerous waste products, increasing the flow of blood through the body, particularly from the heart to the respiratory system.

Check your pulse rate now. Lie quietly on the floor for two

minutes and then count for a full minute. Your pulse may vary from anyone else's but that doesn't matter. Keep a record of it with regular checks as your jogging programme progresses. If it begins to reduce its at-rest rate steadily, you're going well.

9. Getting started

B EFORE WE SET about this business of jogging, there are
three basic injunctions I make frequently and forcefully:

1. Before you jog, see your doctor, explaining what you
want to do and ask for a thorough check-up. There are
things that might affect your ability to jog in complete safety
and you should know before you find out the hard way. You
need a medical clearance first.

2. When you jog, you train. DON'T STRAIN.

3. You can easily run too fast for your benefit. YOU CAN
NEVER RUN TOO SLOWLY.

I called jogging a business because, if you want to continue
to enjoy good health, it is something you have to work at.
But it is not a chore.

Taking your doctor into your confidence first is vital.
Some heart conditions can preclude jogging, some do not.
One plus-60 runner in New Zealand ran several marathons
but he could never get a pre-race medical certificate from the
race doctor because he had a definite heart murmur. He had
to carry a special certificate from his own doctor, who knew
his complaint well and knew that it was not dangerous for
him to run the 26 miles (42 kilometres) at his own pace.
Medical certificates are no longer required for marathons, of
course.

Even when you have become a seasoned jogger, you
should not hesitate to keep in touch with your doctor — for
reassurance and for an added check on your improvement in
general condition.

New Zealand spends about $16 million a year on medical social security. The United States bill for the heart alone was $22 billion in 1973. It seems we try to keep our national health with drugs when we could spend much of the money far more profitably in educating people to take an active interest in their own physical welfare before they get to the stage of needing assistance. If we did, we would not only cut the bill, we would have healthier nations.

We made the point earlier that the sporting life of the average New Zealander and probably many other people, too, ends in the late 20s or early 30s when he or she stops and does nothing strenuous for the next 15 or 20 years. At that point, he or she suddenly finds an overweight problem, the beginnings of blood pressure and that other symptoms are developing which suggest coronary heart disease.

This is why we cannot emphasise enough the importance of consulting your doctor first and clearing yourself medically before you begin the process of getting fit and not fat. You must be sure that you have not already passed the point of no return beyond which sudden physical effort could be damaging.

Your main item in jogging is the shoes you wear. Nothing else is more important. They must be comfortable and well cushioned with a good sole of rubber, particularly beneath the heel. The rubber needs to be semi-resilient. You can drop hard rubber and it won't bounce. You can drop very soft rubber and it won't bounce. Neither is good for your shoes. You need a semi-microcellular rubber which will bounce when it is dropped. This is most important for anyone planning to run or jog a large mileage.

The mere fact that a shoe seems to have a lot of rubber beneath it doesn't mean you will get a lot of protection. The back of the heel must not bite into the achilles tendon and the heel should not be cut away because, if you are running correctly and aerobically, with a heel-to-toe roll, too much fairing will cause jarring at the back of the foot which can affect your ankles, knees, hips and back. It is all right to have a heel that is turned a little as long as there is good rubber right under the heel.

The waffle sole is ideal if you are going to be running on trails or grassy areas but on the road it wears down quickly and there is significant loss of traction. The more sole you can plant on the running surface the greater the traction. Think of the dragster driver — he uses the widest, flattest tyres he can for 100 per cent traction. It is the same with running shoes. The traction loss with waffles is particularly bad on wet roads.

Take care with your selection of shoes. With jogging becoming the way of life for increasing thousands of men and women, the footwear market has been flooded with all kinds of shoes for running, jogging, road and track work. Some are expensive and some are not. Some are excellent and some are next to useless. Some are cosmetically attractive but lack the under-foot protection or the basics of design that ensure foot comfort during prolonged running. Check carefully before you buy and be prepared, on this item, to spend perhaps a little more than you might have planned or think you should have to.

Your shoes should not be too loose — or too tight, either. Your feet will swell when you run and if your shoes are tight you'll have established one of the biggest causes of blisters. The same with socks, if you are going to wear them. Make sure they have no holes or darns which could cause chafing or blistering and make sure they don't bunch up inside your shoes as you run by crawling down under your heels.

The front of the shoes should be just clear of the toes. If the shoe is too long or too big, the joint of the foot where the forepart is widest will be caught back in the waist of the shoe, where it is narrower, and you will get blistering on the inside of the foot.

Some shoes are oversprung. By this I mean that when the shoe is taken off the last it springs flat on the toe instead of staying like a box. This means the upper part will pull down on the toe nails and you will almost certainly lose them.

Many shoes are made on a straight last but your foot is more of a banana shape, which means that you often get pressure points on the outside of the big toe and on the inside of the heel. To control this fault, some shoe makers insert a hard stiffener or counter in the shoe, which then forces the forepart of the foot to overhang the edge of the sole on the outside of the shoe. Since, when you run, your foot tends to want to go to the outside anyway, you end up with the foot being forced right over, causing ankle and knee problems and, probably, the fairly rapid collapse of the shoe. This straight shoe-banana foot mix is the main reason why many runners need orthotics in their shoes in a bid to achieve balance in an unbalanced shoe.

Care of your feet is vital. Do something silly, blister them or bruise them through insufficient padding, and days of training and exercise can be lost. So can the incentive to keep going.

Even the way you lace your shoes is important. The best method is illustrated. Any other lacing tends to create pressure points across the top of the foot, which can become uncomfortable and even painful when your foot swells.

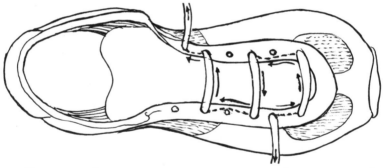

If you can, begin your jogging on grass, unless it is too soft and slushy. Grass is easier on the legs and feet when you set out, particularly if you are a big person carrying a lot of extra weight. The lower limbs are going to do all the harder work and they deserve every consideration you can give them until you have toughened up.

Your foot action is important. You should land nearly flat-footed, heel first and then rolling along the outside of the foot before driving off the toes. Some of you with high arches and tight achilles tendons will possibly need higher heels on your shoes to alleviate tendon strain. Your tendency will be to land on the forepart of the foot, which sets up a resistance against normal traction, almost a braking effect. This is a cause of blistering and, worse, shin splints and calf muscle soreness. The higher heels will help you to get the correct footfall.

Because, in jogging, the forward momentum is not fast, the body's centre of gravity takes longer to get over the lead leg (unlike the sprinter's) and this is why it is best to roll over the foot with a heel-to-toe action. Some people will not be able to run heel and toe and they are advised to run on grass or trail areas where there can be less traction.

The overweight runner may find that his ankles will swell. He can counter this by wearing support bands while he runs and by exercising as much as possible to strengthen the ankles. This is discussed later.

The clothing you wear when you run is less important than the shoes on your feet but heed a few important points. Clothing should be loose-fitting without being annoyingly floppy. Don't let elastic leg bands restrict the thighs and avoid tight waist-bands. Shorts are better than long pants because they give more freedom of movement. The material should be of soft texture to avoid chafing. A loose-fitting sweater or windbreaker is useful when there is rain in the air or a bite in the wind; but you will find that, if you over-dress, you will over-heat and begin tearing garments off before you are very far from home. Choose clothing appropriate for the prevailing conditions. You need the warm clothing after your running to protect you against chills.

The jogger who wants to lose weight fairly quickly in the beginning should wear extra clothing to help in working up a sweat. The higher body temperature takes blood from the working muscles, putting more stress on the heart. Wear clothing which is suitable for the conditions and allows for comfort while you are running. Incidentally, the weight loss through jogging will not be spectacular. What you sweat away is mainly water which will be replaced almost as fast as it runs off.

As we get fit, our bodies feel a new toughness and handle conditions like cold and wet much better. In the early jogging period, woollen socks or protective bands rather than tight elastic bands on your ankles and knee pads will help to keep the cold out of, and the heat in, your joints until they become accustomed to working properly again.

Special bras are available for women today, goretex suits are now made for wear in unusually adverse conditions and, in general, the range of jogging clothing is such that, in whatever climate you run, you should have no difficulty in being properly and comfortably outfitted.

One warning for men: You can suffer chafed nipples from certain materials. Protect them with vaseline or a similar lubricant or cover them with plasters. Chafing which occurs in other areas, such as the crutch and armpits, can also be checked by using lubricant.

Muscle soreness will occur but it is nothing to be upset about and should not deter you from continuing your jogging, as long as you understand what is happening. When we set our guinea-pig joggers going in 1961, some had not run for 20 or 30 years and they were warned they would get sore. So they expected to get sore, they got sore, they continued jogging — and they got over the soreness.

It can even be a healthy sign because some soreness indicates changes for the better are taking place in your body. One cause is the stepped-up flow of blood forcing its way into and opening up capillary beds that have not been used in a long, long time and the rupturing of some muscle sheaths.

Other causes are the accumulation of damaged and used blood cells because your muscles are inefficient in handling waste products and the creation of the oxygen debt because unfit novice joggers lack sufficient haemoglobin, quickly build up restricting lactic acid in the bloodstream and muscles and feel the resulting tenderness. They may also get aches from chest muscles strained by sustained use during heightened breathing.

Giving in to soreness is a mistake. It is a fairly necessary hurdle which has to be crossed and you will get over it faster and with a minimum of discomfort if you become a regular jogger prepared to bear some initial pain.

10. On your way

I F YOU ARE going to do your jogging with a group, don't let it develop into an endurance test or any form of race. Don't be influenced by runners who can move faster than you can. For reasons of which you have no need to be ashamed, others may develop stamina faster and outstrip your progress. Equally, you may be the fast developer and you should not let that lead others astray.

Recognise your own capabilities and stay within them. You have specific reason for jogging and it has nothing to do with proving yourself better than other people or letting them prove they are better. You are not aiming to break the four-minute mile but to regain and maintain good health, vim and vigour — and you won't get them by indulging in races with your neighbours. The process has to be gradual and con-trolled within your own steady state.

If you are the fastest in a group, it won't hurt you to match your pace back to theirs. You can always finish off with an extra turn around the block. The extra distance, in fact, will do you more good than extra speed.

If everyone keeps this in mind, the 30-year-old and 60-year-old can jog together and both benefit equally. If one or both has to stop and walk part of the way, both will still be doing themselves nothing but good. Slower joggers will only go backwards, or down in a heap, if they try to foot it with faster joggers who don't bother to consider comparative capabilities.

I try to encourage everyone to match themselves to the

pace of the slowest but this is not always easy, unfortunately, because of our natural competitiveness. Jogging should be a cooperative, non-competitive, combined exercise in relaxation when packs are running. If it is not, someone in there could be damaging themselves. If that person is you, let them go, and take your own time for your own sake.

No way of exercising is more rewarding than distance running. Ask Halberg and Snell. Ask Barry Magee, long retired from the running which won him an Olympic marathon medal in 1960 and made him one of the world's fastest 10,000 metres runners of his era but still running marathons comfortably under 2:30 though he is now in his mid-40s. Ask any seasoned jogger.

It doesn't take long for anyone to be able to run for half an hour or more at his or her own pace. Joggers will gradually and subconsciously run faster as they become fitter — but not if they attempt to match strides with everyone else.

In April 1981, 2736 people ran a marathon around New Zealand's Lake Rotorua, an annual event which attracted only 16 starters when it began in 1965. Of those participants in 1981, 323 men were in the 40-45 age group, 206 in the 45-50 group, 107 in the 50-54 group, 41 in the 55-59 group and 15 more than 60. A total of 303 women ran and 102 of them were veterans of more than 35 years of age. A total of 2548 finished.

Significantly, the joggers in the field tended to finish better than the open race runners because they were not trying to beat anyone else, only to prove themselves. They had set their targets in time and effort and paced themselves to achieve those targets.

We don't suggest that, when you begin jogging, you have to look to running a 26-mile marathon to prove yourself. It is not necessary for fitness but it does show what simple jogging can achieve when it is fully understood and carefully controlled within the individual's own capacity.

To the novice jogger, beginning basically unfit, we recommend minimal inaugural runs. Out from home for five minutes and then back again running at an even pace. If it takes you more than five minutes to get back from the turning point, you've had your first lesson the hard way. You went out too fast for your condition.

Five minutes may not seem like much of a run but, believe us, when you have run it too fast and you have to get back again over the same distance, it represents a long passage of time.

Anyway, next time, take it easier on the outward leg. Try to spread that even pace over the whole of your run — even if you feel it is little more than a walk. When you can run for 10 minutes without stopping or struggling, try 7½ minutes out and 7½ minutes back again, then 10 minutes each way. Each time you comfortably master one time, add a few more minutes; master them and add some more.

Be patient and you'll be astounded how quickly you can learn to run for half an hour and more — and really enjoy it.

But be warned — and taking the lesson from these pages is much easier than learning it the hard way: Be impatient and you'll take much longer than necessary to achieve a respectable running time. We are quite serious, because we have proved it tens of thousands of times, when we say you could soon find it no trouble to run for an hour, even two hours, if you remember always to keep within your own capabilities so that your jogging is smooth and not strained; if you avoid attempting any effort of time or distance for which you have not undergone a steady build-up.

Depending on your age and condition and application, it could take you from several weeks to several months of patient controlled jogging, of always avoiding breathlessness, of always curbing any inclination to stride out too fast; but whether you get there quickly or slowly, you will get there fit.

Only a few weeks are needed to make you a seasoned jogger who will find it challenging and rewarding to take an extra turn around the block occasionally or add another kilometre or two without anything like the effort an extra 100 metres is likely to be during the first week of jogging.

Psychologically, during this build-up period, it is best to work on a time basis rather than mileage. How long it takes you to run a mile or a kilometre is not important. How long you stay comfortably on your feet is. Comparing your speed with that of a four-minute miler is not jogging. Comparing your 20-minute run with last week's 15-minute run is.

Mileage and time in relationship never become important to jogging unless of course you progress to the semi-competitive field of veterans' group distance races and marathons or club runs.

This is the broad basis of learning to jog. Because it is so essentially simple, it is also fraught with risks — of being impatient and pushing yourself into efforts you're not ready for and which won't do you any good. The benefits you gain from jogging actually come unnoticed; they are not attained by flogging yourself a little harder.

Begin easily, keep going easily. The object is to get the circulation going quietly without creating the oxygen debt that exhausts you and causes muscle soreness. Allow your body plenty of chance to absorb the benefits of the work you are giving it. Do not ever attack jogging like a bull attacking a gate. You have only one competitor to consider in this phase of jogging — the early grave.

Light massage can help in the initial stages and hot baths and Finnish sauna are always beneficial. Unless you are at certain periods of treating some minor injuries, keep your muscles as warm as possible at all times.

The aim is regular running within your own capacities, at least three and up to seven times a week — and this has nothing to do with what your neighbour or your business acquaintance can do. Others may boast of their distances or speed but, if you approach jogging quietly, as they probably did when they began, it won't be long before muscle soreness disappears — and then you're away. The extra mileage, the extra minutes on the feet come naturally; the increase in jogging speed, which is not essential anyhow, comes just as naturally, usually as a pleasant surprise because it happens without any extra effort on your part.

Some of you will suffer longer than others, possibly because of the way you have been living, possibly because you are naturally less athletic in build and weight. If you sit or stand all day without much movement to keep your circulation going, you will feel it for quite a while because you could well be forming a minor oxygen debt during your normal day of inactive work. You have to recognise your degree of preparedness, or unreadiness, to begin jogging and adjust yourself mentally to the task of overcoming your beginner's aches and pains.

The reward of extra stamina comes from conscious work. Other benefits come almost subconsciously. You'll probably smoke fewer cigarettes, take fewer drinks, eat more sensibly. You'll get a new awareness of your physical condition — a more critical appreciation of your own health. You'll begin doing those things that help you to be healthier in everyday life.

We don't believe that people who enjoy smoking and drinking should find it compulsory to stop both completely but, obviously, they would be advised to moderate both habits. Neither makes any contribution to healthier living. Consider it this way: People who don't smoke, drink and exercise will not be as fit as those who do smoke, drink and exercise in reasonable proportions.

Now, having begun this steady build-up, you might wonder if it is necessary to keep on until the end of your days. Do you have to keep on increasing your distance? Simply, it is your choice. But we know that if you train for a year along the lines we suggest and then stop and revert to your former way of living, it would take three or four years more for your pulse rate to fall back to the rate it was before you began training. You can freewheel all that time.

Fifteen to 30 minutes' jogging every day, over a period of 18 months, can double the elasticity and capacity of your arteries. But the degeneration, if the exercise is then stopped, will be many times slower.

Atheroma doesn't become a serious condition overnight. It takes years to grow on you. This means, quite simply, that if you put in a year building your stamina to a high level, you can then relax your efforts and hold that stamina intact with a much reduced programme.

The big thing, if you do taper off, is to aim to have at least one reasonably long jog of, say, an hour or so, every week. But we'll suggest that once you have established the pleasant routine of a jog as part of your daily life, you will be reluctant to abandon or curtail it. You'll find it upsetting to your conscience to begin missing.

Jogging is like banking. The more you put in, the greater the interest. And it is far better to bank a little every day than deposit an hour one day and then nothing more for three or four days. The value of that once-a-week long jog is greatest when you do the regular shorter-time work in between. This is the recognised principle of my training schedule for athletes. The seventh day of every training week — which means 52 weeks a year — is reserved for the long easy jog of 24 to 40 kilometres.

We do not advocate aiming for the marathon distance though many of our joggers have run this event successfully — some of them in incredibly good times for their ages — because they have become so interested in the development of their stamina that they want to see to what lengths they can go.

The longer run once a week will show its value quickly. Because of it, you will come much more rapidly to successive peaks of fitness. You may have to overcome a mental barrier in running for this length of time, particularly if you do your running alone, so we recommend that you do not try it around a track or short circuit — the boredom is bad — but over a selected route that varies the terrain and the scenery.

If this course doesn't lead you back home, ask a member of the family or a friend — if they are not running with you — to bring a car out about 45 minutes after you have left home. By the time you have run that long, the realisation that someone is on the way to pick you up will give you new mental encouragement to look ahead to just how far you are likely to travel before you are overtaken. You'll forget you've been running for so long. But don't try to race on over extra distance.

Once you've successfully jogged a long one, the future long jogs won't be any problem. Quite likely, you'll soon begin to wonder just how far you could go. We've seen it happen so often. Thousands of joggers, for instance, have stepped out to 50 miles (80 kilometres). Millions more realise now that they had never before been fit in the true sense; that they are in better condition now than they were in their twenties, when they could not have hoped to run steadily for three, two or even one hour.

And many of those older and wiser people have noted that, out on the streets and in the parks, they are meeting more and more younger men and women who have also got the message of the daily jog routine.

11. Why strain when you can run

W HY RUN? WHY not work out in a gymnasium with calisthenics or weights training?

We'll put it this way. We are all busy people with limited time. We have got to use that time to the best advantage. We don't want 'keeping fit' to dominate our lives any more than we want them to be dominated by ill-health.

And if you want to prove to yourself what the best advantage is, try this little experiment: Get down on the floor and do some press-ups. Nice, simple things — and we'll give you credit for doing 20 or so, rather than five to 10, before you can no longer get your stomach off the floor. When you get up, your arms and shoulders will be tired but you will not be exhausted and the rest of your body will not feel the effects at all.

Now go outside and run down the road for, say, half a mile. Not far, is it? But now how do you feel? We'll tell you. You'll be leaning on the fence, blowing like a train, feeling as if a red-hot poker had been rammed down your throat, your lungs had been uprooted and your legs turned to rubber. You'll be sweating freely and you'll be wondering if you'll ever get your breath back. That's the way I felt at the age of 27 and my co-author felt at 36.

It hasn't taken you much longer to run down the road than it has to struggle through the press-ups but compare the bodily reactions. The press-ups excessively strained the arm and shoulder muscles, with a slight increase in the pulse rate. The run stirred up the whole body and set the pulse racing.

In that experiment, if you choose to do it, you hit somewhat exaggeratedly on what counts most in fitness and health — the cardio-respiratory system. It has shown that, by jogging, you get at the organs that really matter. You have stimulated the circulation and that is what we are trying to get you to do. Bulging muscles may look fine but they don't do much for you.

Incidentally, while we are on this subject, a special word for women: Jogging or running will not build bulky, bunchy muscles. There are photographs in this book to prove it. The effect is usually the reverse — limbs become finer, more supple, more shapely the more you run.

We will admit that it is more inviting on a wet, cold night to work indoors than it is to get soaked on the street but the minor discomforts of rain and wind are worth the superior results you'll achieve. As long as you keep warm and don't stop moving, you needn't worry too much about colds and chills. As soon as the run is over, get into a hot bath or shower; don't let the sweat on your body and in your clothing get cold on you.

There is even the possibility that, in time, you'll become immune to colds. And it becomes very pleasant to work among sneezing and snuffling people and not experience the illness or fear catching it from someone else.

This is a conditioning a gymnasium will not give you. It is a fact that, not only in jogging but in athletic training, coaches generally did not realise for years the difference between exercise that affects the muscular system and exercise that helps the cardio-respiratory system. They did not appreciate that the cardio-respiratory system is the first and most important target in making anyone fit, to give him or her the stamina, the ability to exercise muscles hard without tiring quickly. It is not a question of building strength first but of giving the cardio-respiratory system the capacity to work under pressure for long periods.

Every time you stand up after a long period of sitting, your heart will work harder. But it has the capacity to work 20 times harder than it normally does and the object of exercise is to lift that normal working level up towards the maximum capacity. The aim is a happy medium which makes the heart work hard enough to begin conditioning the cardio-respiratory system without creating a great oxygen debt.

Jogging involves lifting the body against gravity, an effort which requires the heart to work harder. How hard it works depends on the speed of the running. In jogging, the speed is not great enough to work the heart to excess; it sets up a gentle, steady demand rather than a short, severe one.

The person standing still, lifting weights, is imposing strain but not of the kind that would work the heart, and therefore the cardio-respiratory system, evenly and steadily. The long-distance swimmer is somewhat the same as the runner though the balance of effort is altered because of the reduced weight of the body in the water and the concentration of greater effort in the arms and shoulders.

The bicycle rider, too, is pushing a reduced weight, except when he stands on his pedals to push up hill. As long as he is sitting on the seat, after transferring the weight of his machine from inertia to momentum — from, that is, an opposing force to a helping one — he is being supported against gravity. Same with the person in the rowing boat.

Compared with these other forms of activity, in which the body is either artificially supported or some parts of it are not functioning fully — the rower's legs or the cyclist's arms, for instance — the value of running becomes apparent. It is also the most natural action, requires no special equipment and is available anywhere at any time.

Runners are not only working the cardio-respiratory system, they are giving flexibility to ankles, knees, hips, waist, shoulders, neck, elbows and wrists by the complete and constant movement of every part of the body. All the movements are natural ones for which the body is designed.

We are not knocking other sports, except as they apply to people who seek a form of exercise which will lengthen the full and healthy enjoyment of life at an age when they are beyond most super-active competitive sport.

Every sport requires stamina — and it is now accepted that the one type of exercise that will produce stamina for every sport is controlled running or jogging. Today's coaches and athletes are paying a great deal of attention to the conditioning of the body and the building of stamina before beginning their programmes to refine the required muscular activity and skills peculiar to the sport in which they coach or compete. Even for seasonal sport, conditioning now goes on 365 days of the year, through stamina building backed up by light calisthenics to gently tone the muscles used most in the specific sporting activity.

Then, as the season nears, distance running is tapered off, apart from the occasional freshening jog, and concentration turns to exercises to sharpen the critical muscles. This applies to any sport — tennis, squash, golf, cricket, football, volleyball, you name it. South Africa's Gary Player, who began playing the greatest golf of his long career in his forties, has been a dedicated jogger-calisthenics man to maintain a standard of fitness, reflex action and concentration which overcomes the fact that, physically, he is a small man among power-hitting giants like Nicklaus, Palmer and Trevino.

The stamina-conditioned athletes go into specialised training with a finely tuned cardio-respiratory system. Even the first game of tennis or baseball isn't tiring and they come up fresh for the next one. They are more ready to absorb the benefits of coaching and practical match experience. Jogging isn't just for track and road athletes any more — it is for everyone who wants to play their chosen sport better.

Up to now, most people have passed through life without realising what their true athletic potential is or was. They just didn't attack the serious business of long-term physical development properly. We don't believe that people with a normal pulse rate can know how good they are at any sport until the rate is down to 50 beats a minute or slower, because, until it gets down there, they are not basically fit by today's standards. And if they are not basically fit, how can they concentrate on the finer, more technical abilities of sport?

For example, how can the footballer concentrate on correct handling and passing of the ball if he is puffing and blowing from the previous 20-metre dash? If his lungs are pumping painfully, where is he going to find that extra spurt in an emergency which will get him away from a tackle or block or through a gap to the scoring line?

How are cricketers going to make those extra few runs if they are so tired physically and mentally that they cannot move quickly enough to catch the loose ball or defend themselves against the one that comes in a little sharper than all the others?

How are fencers going to keep going through a succession of pools against progressively stronger opponents if the muscles are beginning to ache and to respond more slowly, if they are so tired that their normal lunge is a split second slower than it could be?

How is the golfer going to have the relaxed control needed for that vital putt or that critical shot to a tightly bunkered green if the muscles are taut and quivering with fatigue?

How often is a person beaten by another with no greater technical skills, perhaps even fewer, simply because they have failed to last the pace as well?

How are you going to maintain your concentration on that business discussion, that intricate technical problem or that critical working drawing if your body is drooping with late afternoon tiredness and your mind is more concerned with getting some rest than with the issue at hand?

The principle of stamina applies to all sports because it stands to reason that the person who stops training out of season goes backward in condition, however slowly. As in business, you either advance or go back and, while you may coast along safely as a jogger on periods of reduced effort or even no effort at all, as an active athlete you cannot afford to in today's highly competitive and training-intensive sports. The day you train, you are gaining ground on the person who is not. Similarly, the day you jog, you are gaining on your main competitor, your own advancing years.

But, let's repeat again, sustained speed running or excessive exercising do not condition the body as effectively as a reasonably steady speed or effort. The former will be constantly building an oxygen debt and the breakdown in the body can become so great that it gets little chance to absorb any real benefit from the effort. But people who exercise regularly within their own capabilities, with a steady but minimal pressure against current mental and physical limits, will be constantly consolidating and slowly adding to the capacity to exercise.

The day you begin to bust yourself and put strain on, you begin to wear your condition down. This is evident in athletes who do a great deal of speed training without first conditioning for stamina. They break their condition down as fast as they build it up. They may reach a peak level of performance fairly quickly but they cannot hold it like the stamina athlete. They peak once and decline. The stamina athlete peaks gradually and then holds it in a controlled series of peaks and plateaus for about as long as they like. The speed merchant becomes mentally sick of exercise because the exercise constantly hurts.

It used to be suggested that our concept of 160 kilometres a week of conditioning running would burn athletes out, because it seemed excessive and therefore was deemed to be harmful. But, at 32, Murray Halberg capped 12 years of top flight international running with his fastest-ever 10,000 metres. Barry Magee can still cruise a marathon in less than 2:30. And the critics didn't understand that my athletes regularly ran 300 kilometres or more a week because they supplemented the basic 160 kilometres with an equal amount of recovery and relaxation jogging.

You may wonder what all this has to do with jogging. It has everything to do with it because these are exactly the principles — if not the mileages — we want you to apply to keep fit. The goal is different but the pathway to it is the same. You don't aim to be faster and stronger than the next person — but won't it be nice to know you'll probably live longer and more happily. You cannot do that by roaring into your jogging like a speed-trained, hare-brained sprinter.

Approach jogging quietly, sensibly and steadily, with an understanding of what makes it work, just as it works in different proportions for the world's best middle and distance runner, and you'll climb to an inevitable and enviable peak of condition. The occasional extra effort you throw in will give the whole conditioning process booster shots to get you there faster.

Once you have reached your first peak, you'll be able to hold it and add to it, like the marathon-trained runner, with remarkably little subsequent effort and a great deal of enjoyment. It's like building a fire on a sound basis — you have to feed it only moderately to keep it blazing. Just take your time about it once you have started. Remember, you have the whole of your life to do it in.

A few words on technique because how you run makes all the difference, and discipline from the beginning will keep the errors out. If you can, keep to reasonably level ground in your initial running. Wait until you loosen up and gain some strength before you tackle the hills. They offer a lot of resistance and, while they're excellent later for giving quick results, they can be demoralising to the beginner. They can pull the legs around too much before they are strong and limber enough to stand full wear and tear; and downhill running can strain unready stomach muscles.

The correct way to run is as simple as the right way to walk. You walk upright, with the torso balanced over the hips, arms relaxed and swinging straight through, the thumbs coming through in line with the insides of the shoulders. That is exactly how you should run.

If you let your hips get back, you bend forward and you cannot get your knees up; if you cannot get your knees up, you shorten stride length and lose stride speed. You cannot land lightly and easily with the correct roll from heel to toe.

Work consciously at running relaxed. Arms, shoulders, neck, upper body should all be comfortable, naturally relaxed, so that no effort is being wasted. Arms should be low and with almost no action because they make no significant contribution to running except to maintain balance.

Your feet should fall almost in a straight line, something you can check by running across a dewy grassland or on a beach. If they are not in line, you could be running out of balance and you are certainly wasting some effort by shifting the body from side to side instead of directly straight ahead. This is not vastly important for the non-competitive runner but, since it is good technique, you should be concerned to master it.

We often get middle-aged runners who complain that they get stuck at a certain running speed, say, 8-minute miles (5-minute kilometres), whether they run three miles (five kilometres) or 20 miles (32 kilometres). They cannot improve that average speed. Usually it is because they are what we call 'sitting in the bucket'. Their legs are always bent; they never run tall or get that driving leg straight. Their hips sit back, which inhibits their knee action. Quite often, too, they throw their arms and upper bodies around too much or tense up and hold them tight. This introduces shoulder roll and they lose forward momentum. They don't let their ankles flex enough, maybe they don't use them at all, so they get no benefit at all from the considerable power that conditioned ankles contain.

Every runner, irrespective of age or sex, owes it to himself or herself to determine to improve running technique because it makes running so much easier and so much more satisfying. Correct technique uses a lot less energy to achieve a lot more; poor technique consumes a lot of energy to achieve little.

So after a sensible warm up jog of 15 minutes or so, get out on a field or track and, using a following wind if possible to reduce resistance, practise running tall, with a high knee lift to achieve long relaxed strides, over 100 metres or so. Try to drive off the back leg and foot but don't force it. You want to try to run at a speed just fast enough to enable you to maintain balance, not at your utmost speed. Give yourself time to think about what you are doing. Then jog 300 metres or so and repeat the whole exercise several times. If it is possible, have someone who knows what to look for watch you in action or get yourself videotaped or filmed. It can be quite a lot of fun apart from the value you get from it.

This kind of workout once or twice a week with up to 10 runs through will quickly help the average jogger to improve technique and also adds a different interest to the development of condition.

Ankle flexibility is of utmost importance. Many runners do not use their ankles as much as they should. They tend to use their feet like wheels, rolling through with a stiff ankle, overlooking the power contained in the reflex kick off the back foot which developed ankle flexion can supply.

Try it. Next time out, use your ankle to exert a quick push off the toe and you'll feel your stride lengthen markedly. Be warned though that, if you continue, you will tire quickly because you have not conditioned for it. An excellent static ankle strengthener is to stand on a step, block, book or brick on the balls of the feet and raise and lower yourself, allowing the heels to touch the ground and then lifting them as high as you can. Several times a day works wonders.

On the running side, using a springing action when climbing hills, or bounding part of the way or running up and down flights of steps or stairs are ideal ankle strengthening and flexing exercises that will help to take you from plodder to efficient jogger and, eventually, if that is what appeals, to competent runner.

These are important exercises for the overweight jogger.

12. Cold morning, cool night or on the way to work

W HEN TO JOG? Because it is an aerobic exercise, you can do it at any time that personally suits you. Some find it better in the morning than at night but they need to remember that the body is going to take some waking up when it crawls out of a warm bed on a cold morning. The pulse rate will be slowed right down and the general condition will resent the idea of forcing the body into a hand-gallop down the road into a cold dawn.

It can make the beginning of the early morning run feel awkward and even uncomfortable until the circulation gets going properly. But, once again, your metabolic system is going to take care of you quite naturally and adjust itself to the practice of early rising and early running. A wake-up cup of tea or coffee can help.

If you can get over that initial inertia and, we warn you, it is far from easy, you'll have no further trouble. For the person who arrives home late from work and, therefore, has a late evening meal, the early morning jog is perhaps most suitable. It is also a great exercise in self-control and discipline.

I prefer to train before the evening meal because it is important to run on a reasonably empty stomach and it is a time of day when the body is fully awake. Late night training is fine, if you have adequately lit and paved roads or paths to run on. But then you have to wait for the evening meal to digest, even two or three hours if you eat heavily. Apart from the discomfort of undigested food in the stomach, it takes up space near your heart and lungs which is needed when those organs expand under the pressure of exercise. Remember, too, that the digestive process occupies the attention of about a third of the body's blood supply. You need all that for exercising.

Many joggers have got around the problem of time by adopting a lunch-time run routine but this needs at-work showering and changing facilities and, preferably, a park or quiet streets to run in. Others run to and from work, which is fine if you can solve the clean, fresh clothing problem, have to cover only a comfortable distance and have showering and dressing facilities at both ends. The decision to abandon the car, bus or train and the umbrella and briefcase for shorts and shoes has to be made in the face of possible early ridicule and scepticism but it is an excellent way of achieving that vital exercise without interfering too much with spare time — and, like all joggers faced with the mockery of non-jogging acquaintances, you have that built-in superiority of knowing that what you're doing is what they should be doing and they are the losers.

Really, when you jog is when it is the most convenient and it is governed by your individual circumstances. All we can say is that any time is jogging time. We know of one country town dweller in New Zealand who gets up at 3.00 am and runs for up to two hours on the country roads because he begins work early, the traffic is almost non-existent — and he likes it.

And if prime ministers and presidents can find the time ... ?

13. Trouble shooting

F ROM TIME TO time, like any athlete, you are going to run into problems of varying kinds. None, if you have that clean bill of health medically to begin with, is likely to be serious or insurmountable, though some may interrupt your running programme.

For instance, Clarence deMar, the man the Americans called 'Mr Marathon' — he ran his first race in 1909 and his last in 1957, at the age of 68, and totalled more than 1000 long distance races and 100 marathons — was operated on for cancer and fitted with a colostomy. It did not stop him from marathon running. His death had nothing to do with his heart; it was found that his left coronary had a core four times bigger than normal and doctors who examined him after he died concluded he could never have died of coronary thrombosis.

A Swede who continued running marathons in his seventies left his body to science and was found to have a vascular system which was completely clear except for a slight atheroma near the heart. Heart disease did not kill him, either.

But runners have other, lesser problems and you should know something about them.

Stitch: This can be caused by the jarring effect on the diaphragm or stomach muscles which are not supple enough to take the strain of increased pressure from expanded and faster-working heart and lungs and therefore throw pressure on the ligaments which connect the diaphragm to the skeletal frame. This is a pain which hits you in running but stops as soon as you stop. It can also begin again as soon as you go on. Downhill running, when you stretch those muscles because you lean back more, is also a stitch-producing activity.

Loosening and suppling exercises help. One of the most simple and effective is to put your hands on the edge of the dressing table, place your feet well away from it and then chest the table edge, arching your back as far as possible. About ten of these a day will take care of stitch. Sit ups — with your legs bent to avoid lower back strain — back-bending and hip rotation are also important exercises. Remember, the exercises must be felt in the muscles under the rib cage.

Sore Muscles: These emerge from time to time and in various places. People who run on the balls of their feet and cannot get their heels down first when they are jogging are more likely to have muscle trouble than those who run heel-to-toe. Blisters, damaged toe nails, metatarsal damage and shin splints are all possible injuries, usually through the stretching and pulling about of the muscle sheaths and minor fibre ruptures.

You can get over the basic sore muscle problem by running on sand or grass until the tendons in your legs supple up and until you have mastered the correct foot fall. Building up the heels of your shoes can also help.

Keep an eye on those shoe heels at all times and don't let them wear down too far before you rebuild them. A millimetre or two of wear immediately alters the angle at which your foot hits the ground and can put strain on ankles, knees, hips and lower back.

Achilles Tendon: Ball-of-the-feet runners are susceptible here and so is every beginner until the muscles and tendons are supple and strong. This is one reason why you should stay off the hills until you have reached a good level of muscle condition. Use exercises daily to stretch them.

Hamstring: A problem caused by leg-speed running with muscles and sinews that are not stretched and conditioned equally, usually because the quadricep muscles are stronger than the hamstring muscles. The sheathing around muscle fibres breaks down and the fibres themselves can be torn. It can happen if you don't warm up gently; it can happen even if everything is done properly because of the stress of using these muscles for long periods and a slow breaking down of muscle tissues. Well-toned athletes can pull muscles under the most perfect conditions.

Recovery, particularly from achilles tendon damage, is never easy. Conventional treatment consists of ice packs applied immediately to reduce internal bleeding around the injury area, heat treatment or gentle massage two or three days later, once the injury is confined, water therapy and so on — all of which can take a month. One American doctor has decided that the best method is to immobilise an injured tendon by encasing it in plaster for two weeks. Well, it is quicker.

When you do pull a muscle, you can put your finger accurately on the spot. There will be internal bleeding there which you must stop, so avoid heat or manipulation for three days. In that time, ice or cold water is the required treatment. By then, scar tissue will have formed around the injured area and heat treatment or massage will then help to get rid of the excess blood around the tissue and stimulate food supplies to the injury zone.

Incidentally, in all cases of injury, it pays to go to a physician rather than treat yourself. You could make the damage worse.

Shin Splints: These are membrane ruptures between the muscle and the bone and often arise from the jarring of downhill running or over-striding. You can counter over-striding by building up the front of your shoes a little and you should always be careful when running downhill to shorten stride and take it easy.

Water therapy, cold packs and eventual heat treatment help this injury. Water therapy — using a kickboard in a tepid pool or simulating the running action while treading water — is invaluable for all leg injuries.

Joint Injury and Bone Wear: These are invariably caused

by poor shoes with insufficient buffering to prevent jarring on hard surfaces. Without plenty of bouncy rubber between you and the ground, the shock of each stride is felt over a wide area of the body and problems can arise in unexpected places. The only remedy is total prevention with good shoes.

All this advice gets back to one point — it is easier to prevent than it is to cure. Consider in advance what you are doing with your body and give it all the protection it needs, such as well-soled shoes, warm clothing when it is needed and carefully avoiding excessive strain and over-striding.

If you have muscle aches and pains from the previous day's run, take it easy. Get on sand or grass, slow right down and shuffle the discomfort away. This is better than trying to maintain normal speed or putting your feet up and waiting for the aches to go away.

14. Temperatures, electrolytes and you

Y OUR BODY TEMPERATURE varies throughout your body. You lose heat by physical processes and physiological factors which cool the blood as it flows near the skin and provide water for cooling the skin by vaporisation.

In cold air, the blood vessels in the skin contract to diminish heat loss; in high temperatures, or when exercise produces extra body heat, the blood vessels dilate. More perspiration is secreted and you lose more heat through evaporation. The more you exercise, the more blood flows through the outer skin area and the more you perspire.

Strenuous exercise, like sustained jogging, sets up a demand for more blood to feed the muscles and sends more to the skin for cooling. The warmer the atmosphere, the greater the demand.

This pressure can at times exceed the capacity of the heart to increase cardiac output, causing nausea, dizziness and even heat-stroke. These are effects unlikely to be experienced in a normal jogging programme but you need to be aware of them if you step up your programme towards the marathon-running distances.

If you are not accustomed to strenuous exercise in the heat, you risk this sequence of consequences:

Heat cramps, through excessive loss of electrolytes and water, which leads to neuromuscular breakdown;

Heat exhaustion, through circulatory inadequacy caused

by dehydration;

And, at the worst, heat-stroke, a condition serious enough to be fatal because the temperature-controlling centre of the brain becomes deranged.

If you live in a hot area, you need to accustom yourself to running in the heat by carefully controlling and lengthening the duration of your exercise periods in the heat. This steadily improves the circulation of the blood to the surface of the skin, where the small skin arterioles are developing, for cooling. Try always to train on a route on which you can get water at regular intervals or have someone supplying you during the run. The steady intake of water is vital.

Marathon runners are often required to compete in hot conditions in which body temperatures rise to extremes and dehydration is excessive. They can handle these conditions if they have trained in similar conditions; if they have not, they rarely finish or, if they do, are in a distressed state for some time afterwards.

Jim Peters' marathon run in the 1954 Empire Games in Vancouver is probably the classic and most-quoted example of a fine runner who came close to death through dehydration and circulatory failure because he was not prepared for the hot conditions in which the race was run.

If you are a regular sauna user, you will recall that you probably began by feeling very hot and even faint in about 80°C but, after a few weeks, could take temperatures up to 120°C without discomfort. The temperature-regulating mechanism of the body is quite efficient — but you still cannot take complete liberties with it.

I had an effective cure for the heat's effects during my marathon-running days. Instead of using the customary sponge at the feeding stations, I would up-end a whole bucket of water over myself. The cooling effect was almost instantaneous and I could run on freely to the next station and the next bucket of water. I found, too, that in cool weather I could run a marathon 10 to 15 minutes faster than on hot days, which indicated the degree to which the body metabolism is taxed by heat.

If you're hoping to lose weight as part of your fitness programme, don't pile on extra clothing on hot days. You'll lose a lot of water and minerals but, because you limit the amount of training you can do by the clothing you wear, you won't be burning as much fat as you would if you wore less, kept your body temperature down and ran longer and faster. In fact, a few hours after your run, you'll have replaced most of the liquid you lost. It is fat you have to burn off and that goes with distance and speed.

Heavy clothing, because it raises your body temperature, also draws more blood from the working muscles to the skin for emergency cooling. This also helps to limit your running and, because as large a volume of running as possible is necessary for cardiac efficiency, you're losing out yet again.

In high temperatures, you can run steadily for an hour or more as long as the humidity is also reasonably high, because the moisture you expire remains on the skin and assists with cooling. In low humidity, evaporation is faster and contributes to dehydration.

Again, I proved this theory on myself. I ran in Tucson, Texas, in 38°C and less than 20 per cent humidity. I lasted about 20 minutes. But in Maracaibo, Venezuela, I trained easily for an hour a day. The temperature was always between 39 and 50°C but the humidity was nearly 90 per cent and I was always wet with perspiration and suffered no ill effects.

The opposite applies if you are training in sub-zero temperatures. If there is moisture in the air when the temperature is between 20 and 40°C below zero, training is almost impossible because you risk icing your lungs. But, if the humidity is below 20 per cent, you can train for hours, provided you are well protected.

The Finns trained comfortably in these conditions by wearing two track suits — a suedette outer one which prevented cold air penetration and an inner one which allowed warm air trapped inside the suedette to pass through so that you ran in a cushion of warm air — a woollen hat, muffler, gloves and socks. Only their cheeks were exposed.

So remember the formula: When the temperature is high, the humidity needs to be reasonably high; when the temperature is low, the humidity needs to be low. If any other combination prevails, be careful and limit your jogging.

If you jog in a warm climate or if you perspire freely, you'll need to replace the minerals as well as the water you lose. It is important to maintain blood balance. The simple remedy is a mineral replacement programme, easily followed by taking an electrolyte preparation. There are several on the market and any which provides calcium, potassium and magnesium is suitable. You need take only about half the recommended dosage to make sure you put back what you lose during exercise and do not necessarily regain from your normal food.

Do not specially take salt drinks or tablets. You get all the salt you need from what you sprinkle on your food and from the electrolyte drink. Salt deletes potassium from the body and potassium is the mineral that protects against hyperthermia. The tablets can cause nausea and gastric irritations and, if you overdose, the excess can be retained in the tissues and blood stream and lead to high blood pressure and hardening of the arteries. There is a limited risk in a well-conditioned body but there is no need to take it at all.

The excellent thing about the electrolyte preparations, which become more valuable an aid as you climb into higher mileages, is that you are virtually drinking back sweat — except that the taste is better.

We will look more closely at the mineral replacement facts later to explain why these are important as part of your happy jogging programme. Meantime, there are one or two other problems of which you should be fully aware.

Hypothermia: Anyone can suffer from this, particularly people running in areas or conditions to which they are not accustomed. There have been too many deaths already to dismiss it as a freak chance. The main problem is that hypothermia is affecting you before you know it and it can then be too late. Three young men died within minutes near Wellington recently when they went for a training run in the bush and encountered a sudden sharp drop in temperature accompanied by a cold wind and rain. They were lightly clad and almost immediately in difficulties from which they could not recover, because no-one was there to help them.

The human body is a machine which works at 37°C. The outer areas can get much colder but the vital organs must stay at that constant temperature. If, in cold, wet and windy conditions, the core begins to cool and the cooling is not immediately checked, you will suffer mental deterioration, loss of co-ordination, unconsciousness and total failure of breathing and circulation. Within 30 minutes of the first symptoms, you can be dead.

Check the progressive warning signs: Tiredness, cold or exhaustion; lack of interest, lethargy; clumsiness, stumbling or falling; slurring speech, difficulty in seeing; irrational behaviour; obvious distress; the cessation of shivering, despite the cold; collapse and unconsciousness; coma.

It sounds unreal and a sense of unreality is one of the warning signs. If you feel any of the early symptoms while you are running in cold, wet and windy weather or note them in a companion, you must act immediately to prevent further heat loss, begin rewarming and try to prevent loss of consciousness. Do not bash on and hope for the best because that can cause the rapid onset of more serious stages. You must get out of the wind, get dry clothing, warm drinks and, essentially, send for expert help.

The best advice, of course, is to be adequately equipped with clothing to protect you against a sudden fall in conditions. Bear in mind that heat loss from the head is high — a fact often overlooked.

Hypocapnia (hyperventilation): You can over-breathe and blow off too much carbon dioxide. This gas is the stimulus to breathe and, if the level in the blood drops, it can cause biochemical changes which lead to giddiness, pins and needles, rapid beating of the heart and a feeling of dread. Breathing may stop and the victim may feel no desire to take a further breath. Because no more oxygen is taken in, the level of this gas reaching the brain drops and this can lead to loss of consciousness.

Then, as the level of carbon dioxide produced by the tissues builds up again, the breathing resumes and the victim regains consciousness. If you sense someone is experiencing this unpleasant phenomenon, the best thing you can do is make him slow down his breathing or breathe in and out of a paper bag which will force him to re-breathe his own carbon dioxide.

Fortunately, jogging creates a surplus of carbon dioxide. Even the outpouring of lactic acid into the blood, by decomposing bicarbonate, lifts the output of carbon dioxide so the chances are you will never be confronted with this quite alarming condition.

15. The things we need

S UGAR HAS LONG been rejected as an item of diet and many have labelled it a strong contributory factor in coronary heart disease — without, we should add, a great deal of support. Many people who laughingly call it 'the white death' still heap it into their coffee and tea. But the evidence against sugar has been accumulating steadily and, through the influence of T. L. Cleave and others in their book *Diabetes, Coronary Thrombosis and the Saccharine Disease,* convincingly.

They suggest a time relation exists between increased consumption of sugar and the marked increase in the incidence of certain diseases. The subject was taken up by Dennis Burkitt who, after years of surgical practice in South Africa, gained a reputation for his work on the type of cancer now named after him. He returned to the staff of the Medical Research Council to examine some surprising differences in the type of disease encountered in the African and European communities and the increase of some previously uncommon diseases in western societies.

He noted that our civilisation has diseases which were not known until a century ago and are not found in domestic animals. Typical of these are alimentary tract disorders, including one disease which takes the form of pea-sized bulges in the colon and today is the most common disease of the large intestine, found in a third of all people over 40 and in two-thirds at 80.

Benign tumours of the same area have been found in a

third of those over 20 and the large intestine has become, after the lung, the most common site of and cause of death from cancer.

Varicose veins affect from 10 to 17 per cent of all adults and would affect more than half of the urbanised western world if they lived long enough. Thrombosis or clot formation in the deep veins of the legs, associated with a slowing of the blood flow through them, complicates up to a third of surgical patients over the age of 40. An associated condition, haemorrhoids, is found in half of those over 50.

Burkitt attributes all of this to a change in dietary habits, particularly to an increased consumption of refined carbohydrates, chiefly as sugar and white flour, with a corresponding reduction in the fibre content of the residues in the large intestine. He estimates that content is only a fifth of what it was before our present bland diet became general.

Consequently, bowel contents are harder, their transit time is prolonged and more pressure is exerted on the walls of the bowel. The overloaded colon presses on the main venous channels and obstructs the return flow of blood from the lower limbs.

Cleave's ideas are in keeping with Burkitt's. As the intake of refined sugar and starch has increased, the eating of food with fibrous residues has decreased. The excess consumption of energy in refined foods has led to obesity; diabetes follows the rapid absorption of digested carbohydrates; and overloading makes demands on the pancreas for the insulin needed for their conversion to energy.

This is somewhat of an over-simplification but it is difficult to see what other factors could have played as significant a part in the development of these abnormalities.

We need the carbohydrates, of course, and the best sources are the grains, potatoes and so on. If you want more, honey, a fructose without bulk, will give you all the blood sugars you need for longer runs without any complications. It is pure energy and because of that it can be taken quite soon before the start of a run without causing problems.

We are often told that salt is necessary for life but Dr Benjamin Rush studied American Indians and found them to be as healthy as Stefanson found the Eskimos and as Bartholomew found the people of interior China. The common factor — none of them ate salt.

Salt in small doses does act as a stimulant; in large doses, it is an embalming fluid. Nutritionist Dr Mary Schwarz Rose, in *Foundations of Nutrition*, declares that the amount of sodium chloride taken in the form of common salt is far in excess of human requirements for either sodium or chlorine, both elements so widely distributed in food materials that there is little likelihood of a shortage of either.

In small doses, salt is immediately eliminated from the body through sweat and urine. In larger doses, it is retained in the body tissues and blood stream, resulting in a state of hyperchloremia.

Eating inorganic salt is a bad habit. Let the plants synthesise sodium chloride into an organic form in their leaves, fruits, roots and stems and eat it that way.

Other stimulants, like coffee, tobacco, alcohol and morphine, can also become concentrated in the blood and body tissues. These, too, can cause violent upsets to the nervous equilibrium as a result of disruption of the correct chemical balance in the body.

So, if we don't need all these things, what do we need? Here are some essentials:

Calcium: Your body contains about 3 lbs (1½ kg) of calcium, more than any other mineral. Most is in your bones and teeth but the remaining one-tenth of one per cent is equally vital. Without it, your muscles would not contract. The mechanism that regulates that small but important amount of calcium is so precise that, if the amount drops a microgram or two too low, calcium is immediately taken from the bones to replace it.

You can unknot cramps, including menstrual cramps, by taking extra calcium. It can often relieve minor back ache and lessen arthritic pain. If you have a lead problem — and just about everyone does who lives in or near a modern city or motorway — a high level of calcium in your diet will help. Calcium stops the absorption of lead.

Exercise has been found to decrease the amount of calcium

lost which is why people who stop exercising as they grow older wind up with weak bones, riddled with holes, which signal their presence most markedly in the humped, curved back of old age.

Protein forces calcium from the body; if you get 100 grams of protein a day in your diet (a typical amount for many westerners), you also need 1000 mg of calcium a day to maintain bone strength (which is not a typical amount for most westerners).

Three glasses of milk a day will provide that amount — all dairy products are packed with calcium — but, because milk also adds fat and calories, it might be best to get it from a supplement. One excellent source is bone meal. Sardines and salmon (with bones), collard or turnip greens and tofu are other valuable sources.

Magnesium: When 200 insomniacs took 500 mg of magnesium a day, they slept at night and their anxiety and tension during the day decreased. Magnesium is a natural tranquilliser: it quiets jumpy muscles as well as nerves. It also is needed for the digestion of protein, fat and carbohydrates and disposes of body odour.

And exercise takes it out of you. Hours-long endurance activity drains it away. So, as a jogger, you must conscientiously think of putting it back.

Magnesium also prevents and has cured kidney stones (the dose was 500 mg a day) and, from autopsies, researchers have found that heart attack victims had 22 per cent less magnesium in their heart muscles than people dying from other causes.

White flour has 28 per cent less magnesium than whole wheat. Canned corn has 60 per cent less than fresh corn. Puffed oats have 33 per cent less than whole oats. Some chemical additives used to keep frozen vegetables green destroy magnesium completely.

Good magnesium sources are whole grains, soybeans, nuts, green leafy vegetables, fruits and blackstrap molasses; but best is dolomite, a preparation from powdered dolomitic limestone, which delivers both magnesium and calcium in the exact proportions nature intended. Whatever, aim for 350 to

500 mg a day.

Potassium: Athletes who don't sweat don't need extra potassium; but those who do and take salt tablets need double doses. Dr James Knochel, a professor at the University of Texas Southwestern Medical School, found that 50 per cent of people hospitalised for heat stroke after intense exercise were potassium-depleted. He found many had taken salt tablets, which forced potassium out of the body and, added to the loss through sweating, lined them up for severe potassium deficiency — nausea, muscle weakness, cramps, irritability and, finally, total collapse.

You don't need to replace salt lost in sweat but you do need to replace the potassium. If anything, you're probably better off sweating the salt away because most of us have too much salt and too little potassium in our diets. Food processing is, again, a major culprit.

Top potassium sources are bananas (a medium-sized banana has 500 mg), oranges, tomatoes, cabbage, celery, carrots, grapefruit, apples, beans and fish.

Vitamins: Much of the following material is drawn from William Gottlieb, senior editor of *Prevention* magazine, writing in *Women's Sport* magazine, who points out that nutrition still is a controversial science, not an exact one and that every 'expert' you ask for advice will probably give you something confusingly different from anyone else.

Gottlieb, who spent four years 'living' vitamins and examining every new study, advance and opinion in the field of nutrition, is convinced of the need to take vitamins.

He says: 'You need to take vitamins if you live in a smoggy city. If you train day after day in the sun. If you eat sugar. If you have an allergy. If you load up on carbohydrates before a race. If you bruise easily. If you're about to compete. To be at the top of your form — in sports and in life — vitamins are a must.'

The body's every action is energised and controlled by enzymes. They are responsible for the steady beat of your heart, your digestion, your breathing and every movement you make — and vitamins are a chemical part of those enzymes which, if removed, would cause the enzymes to stop working.

Vitamin A keeps your skin smooth, your vision sharp, your immune system strong and your anti-stress mechanisms in order. Mostly, we don't get enough because we lean towards fast foods instead of fresh fruit and vegetables. Carrots, sweet potatoes, spinach, apricots and cantaloupe, for instance, contain a substance called betacarotene which, unless destroyed by overcooking, changes to vitamin A in the body. There are 16,000 IU in a cup of cooked carrots. The most concentrated source, of course, is fish liver oil. If you take vitamin E with A, the body's ability to use the A jumps sixfold.

Vitamin B1 is one of the B-complex vitamins and they are usually found together. B1 is thiamine which helps the body turn carbohydrates into glucose which fuels the brain and the muscles. So, if you load up on carbohydrates, add 5 mg of thiamine to help turn them to energy. Like all the B-complex vitamins, what you don't use is excreted, so you cannot over-dose. Thiamine and coffee and alcohol don't mix.

Green leafy vegetables, whole grains, beans, nuts and seeds are thiamine-rich. So are brewer's yeast, wheatgerm and liver.

Vitamin B2 (riboflavin) is good for the eyes and the digestion, tiredness, nerves and lack of appetite. You get it from broccoli and asparagus, milk and cheese, almonds, liver and any whole grains.

Vitamin B3 (niacin) is estimated to fire at least 40 biochemical reactions in the body; the most important involves the red blood cells which carry oxygen to all parts of the body. The last stage in their journey is through the capillaries, the fine networks that you as joggers develop steadily. The red blood cells line up single file in the capillaries and march in; they don't block up because each has a negative electrical charge which forces them apart. Niacin keeps them charged for you. It's in turkey, tuna, peanuts and beef liver.

Vitamin B6 (pyridoxine), which is almost wiped out in processed foods, is a must for the synthesis of serotonin, a brain chemical that regulates memory, helps get rid of acne and soothes many menstrual and pregnancy problems. From lean meats, fish, fresh fruits and vegetables (particularly bananas), nuts, buckwheat, soybeans and wheatgerm.

Vitamin B12 (cobalamin) works on the central nervous system. A deficiency causes fatigue, irritability and some degree of numbness in your limbs. Liver is the best source but any animal product will do.

Vitamin C prevents or cures colds, detoxifies nicotine, alcohol or cancer-causing pollutants, protects against hay fever, increases the ability to exercise in heat. An excess does not, as once feared, cause kidney stones; excess in the urine, in fact, prevents kidney or bladder infections. It comes from all fresh citrus fruits, green peppers, parsley, broccoli and, surprisingly, for most people from potatoes. But not potato chips; they have lost 75 per cent of their vitamin C.

Vitamin D does one job, essential for joggers: It allows the body to absorb calcium, which regulates muscle contractions (like your heartbeat) which makes it important enough. You get very little vitamin D by eating. Sunlight turns a chemical in your skin into vitamin D, which is technically a hormone.

Vitamin E has come to be known as the sex hormone because early researchers found it increased fertility in rats. But improving your sex life is one of the few things vitamin E does not do. It does improve glycogen storage, giving you more fuel for endurance sports; it does improve the tone and strength of your muscles; it does protect cells from oxidation, so that means it probably lengthens life because many scientists theorise that ageing is caused by oxidation.

Processed foods are vitamin E weaklings. Whole wheat bread has seven times more than white bread does, brown rice six times more than white. Find a supplement that has at least 200 IU.

Orotates: The greatest proportion of an oral dose of most minerals does not reach the bloodstream or the target cells so the search has been constant for improved forms of mineral transportation. Orotates promise the best breakthrough for mineral therapy in decades, says Dr Robert Buist, a leader in Australia in the field of preventive medicine and natural therapies.

Orotates are the mineral salts of vitamin B13 combined

with minerals. They are, in general, a non-toxic and highly efficient way of delivering a selected mineral to parts of the body which most need it.

Orotic acid is an organic molecule found in milk whey and synthesised in our bodies from an amino acid called aspartic acid. In the body, it has three main functions: As an integral part of our DNA and RNA, the molecules which mastermind and initiate the body's entire growth and development; in the breakdown of sugar foods to form the energy for bodily functions; and as a bond with calcium, magnesium, potassium and other minerals to take them directly and quickly to the parts of the body where they are needed. This is not the place for a detailed discussion of orotates but it is evident that if you can obtain your mineral supplements in orotate form you are going to derive more immediate and greater benefit from those minerals as instant replacements for whatever your exercising is taking out of you.

Stress: We are back to this subject because it is one of the growing problems of today's fast-moving, constantly changing, high-pressured way of life. American research has found that up to 10 per cent of the population will score in the depressed range on standard depression questionnaires at any one time. National Institute of Mental Health figures indicate that non-psychiatric physicians treat about 60 per cent of patients with psychiatric disorders and refer less than 10 per cent to psychiatrists.

About 80 per cent of the estimated 50,000 American suicides a year are committed by individuals who are depressed. Depressed people are more likely to die of heart disease and infections.

Four Wisconsin people, Drs John Greist and Marjorie Klein, associate professors of psychiatry at the University of Wisconsin, Roger Eischens, a running therapist, and Dr John Faris, a private physician, joined forces when they all noted that their own momentary 'blues' disappeared while they were running. Others reported similar experiences and a lessening of depression generally since they began running.

They set up a programme and here are some of the results: Eleven of 67 normal college faculty members who scored in the depressed range on a specific scale took part in a six-week physical activity study. At the end of the study, each of the 11 had increased physical fitness and no longer had 'depressed' scores. None of the other 56 scored in the depressed range, either.

Of 167 college students who exercised three times a week for eight weeks, doing either wrestling, tennis, varied exercises, jogging or softball, the joggers showed the greatest reduction in depression scores. The softball players and six who did not exercise showed no change.

The team then randomly assigned 13 men and 15 women to either running or one of two kinds of individual psychotherapy. They were all between 18 and 30, complained of depression as their major problem, found their depression interfered with important activities. Ten patients began the running assignment. They ran from 30 to 45 minutes at a comfortable pace three times a week, often with a running therapist, and conversation during the runs concentrated on running technique and associated factors, never on depression.

At the end of ten weeks, two of the ten had dropped out — one left town and the other found running more than he had bargained for when he feigned his way into therapy treatment — and six had recovered from their depression. Since then, other depressed people have recovered through a running programme.

Why it seems to work is a matter of some scientific conjecture but factors which could have influenced the apparent improvement are the sense of success and mastery at becoming a runner against reported drop-out rates for beginning joggers of between 30 and 70 per cent in the first six weeks because of over-straining and consequent failure; the use of patience and the output of regular effort until running becomes a habit; the discovery of the capacity for change in physical health, appearance and body image; the distraction of new bodily sensations; a form of addiction which replaces neurotic defences and habits like smoking, drinking and over-eating; and so on.

One argument advanced by the team: 'At a time when

health costs are rising at alarming rates (at least double the national rate of inflation), it is clearly desirable to identify less costly treatments which provide equal benefits. When a treatment provides better results at lower cost than other treatments in use, that represents a virtually unique situation in medicine.

'Running with a therapist for ten weeks after a screening electro-cardiogram and exercise treadmill test cost less than $15 in our setting. Once-weekly psychotherapy for ten weeks would cost $500 in our community. For individuals who can treat themselves by running without a therapist, the cost becomes that of screening for hidden cardio-vascular weakness or damage before beginning the treatment.'

16. Endurance and the ageing process

D R JOHN L. BOYER, of the San Diego State College's Human Performance Laboratory, has considerable experience in assessing the fitness of United States service personnel and has also spent several years studying participants in the U.S. Masters track and field championships. We quote here from an address he gave at one of the Masters' meetings:

'We now know that ageing is a condition called atherosclerosis, a fatty deposit on the walls of the arteries, which carry blood to the heart, brain, kidney, legs and other important parts of the body. This condition restricts the supply of oxygen and other cellular nutrients, causing the death of cells which are replaced by scar tissue. Just what does exercise do to your heart and blood vessels?

'First, exercise trains the heart muscle just as exercise trains and improves any muscle. It strengthens the muscle fibres of the heart and this makes it a more efficient organ. What kind of exercise does this best?

'Endurance exercise is best to improve the strength of the heart muscle. That is why running, jogging, swimming, cycling or any endurance work is so good. It makes the heart stronger. To support this improved muscle there must be improved circulations — the formation of new vessels and the dilation of existing vessels to improve the blood flow to the muscle fibres of the heart. Thus there is an actual increase of blood to the heart itself with exercise by this collateral system.

'Secondly, exercise increases the size of the heart, just as exercise increases the size of any muscle. This increases the output of blood by the heart with each heart beat. Since the heart is a volume organ, the size and capacity of the heart are very important. The better the volume capacity, the better the stroke volume and cardiac output with each beat.

'Thirdly, exercise decreases the resting heart rate ... a slow resting heart is more efficient. Rates below 70 are optimal.

'An additional benefit of exercise is that it tends to lower the blood pressure. A fourth benefit is called the peripheral benefit. This means that the collateral vessels are also increased to other muscles of the body. This gives another reserve capacity and increases the overall efficiency of the cardio-vascular system.

'A fifth benefit is in the body weight and metabolic area. How much body fat one has compared to lean body mass (muscle) is more important than overall body weight. Optimally, one should have only 10 to 15 per cent of one's weight as body fat. Most sedentary western men have 25 to 30 per cent body fat. Exercise helps to convert the body fat to lean muscle mass.

'Bone metabolism is also improved with exercise. There is an increase of both bone density and bone strength.

'It is easy to see now why running (actually alternating walk and jog) is used as the exercise rehabilitation for cardiac patients. Jogging is an ideal form of endurance exercise. It can be done anywhere and at any time and without any equipment. It does everything for the heart that exercise can do.

'As far as competitive sports for men over 40 are concerned, more than three years' experience with the Masters' meets indicates that it is just great for the trained, conditioned year-round, middle-aged adult. I think competition could be disastrous for the middle-aged man who tries to get ready for competition in a short period of time. This probably is one of the most important points of my talk. Competitive sports for men over 40 are fine provided year-round conditioning and cardio-vascular fitness are maintained.

'In regard to disabilities as the result of strenuous exercise, the same principles apply whether you are 20 or 40. The more fit you are, the less chance you have of an injury.

'The results of our study of participants in the first U.S. Masters track and field championships were about as predicted. They were in the upper echelon of adult fitness levels. In particular, the endurance runners, middle distance and beyond, were outstanding. Some of the field event participants, though in great muscular shape, could have improved their cardio-vascular condition.

'After three years of competition, you might be interested to know that we have had no serious medical problems of any kind. As a matter of fact, at this meet we have had fewer musculo-skeletal problems than at the last A.A.U. national meet held at the same stadium.'

17. No drugs, no surgery, no hardening of the arteries

H ARDENING OF THE arteries — atherosclerosis — kills more than 872,000 Americans a year through heart disease, the nation's No. 1 killer, and strokes. But two separate research programmes reversed the deterioration of the clogged, fat-encrusted arteries of heart patients and led the director of one team, Nathan Pritikin, of the Longevity Research Institute in Santa Barbara, California, to declare: 'It's a revolutionary breakthrough — millions of lives can be saved.'

Both programmes were based on low-cholesterol and low-fat diets *plus controlled exercise*. Pritikin said: 'We proved in 5 out of 12 patients, or 42 per cent, that advanced hardening of the arteries can be reversed.'

Dr David H. Blenkenhorn, of the cardiology section of the University of Southern California in Los Angeles: 'We have seen improvement in 9 out of 40 atherosclerosis patients, or nearly 25 per cent.'

All patients in both programmes already had heart disease when they entered the groups. Many had suffered heart attacks. Some of them could barely walk.

In the five-months LRI programme, patients receive a diet of 10 per cent protein, 10 per cent fats and 80 per cent complex carbohydrates, plus walking exercise of five to 20 miles a day. Cholesterol intake is reduced to nearly zero. The USC programme, though similar, is less severe.

Cardiologist Dr John Kern, clinical instructor at the University of California Medical School at Irvine, who helped the LRI programme, said: 'I was amazed at the results ... it wasn't long before the patients, many of whom could hardly walk before the study, were even running long distances.'

One patient was Leon Perlsweig, a 55-year-old Los Angeles attorney. He said: 'I was ready for heart surgery. I had trouble walking from the back of my house to the front. When the doctors told me I'd soon be able to run a mile — without surgery — I didn't believe them. Now I can run seven or eight miles a day.'

American Heart Association president Dr John T. Shepherd: 'It's the first sign of optimism that heart disease can be licked.'

You can lick it long before you become a heart programme patient. Begin jogging now.

18. Diet and the jogger

C ERTAIN BASIC RULES of diet play a crucial role in the
capacity of every athlete to perform better and to endure
training. For example, studies are constantly showing the
importance of carbohydrates in athletic performance.

Chronic exhaustion is related to muscle glycogen depletion
and a diet of 60 per cent carbohydrate has been found
inadequate to restore muscle glycogen to pre-training levels.
It has been shown that it takes about five days to restore glycogen supplies through carbohydrate ingestion; that a large
store of muscle glycogen is needed for continued and effective
muscle work.

Carbohydrates can be stored effectively. One method is to
deplete the glycogen in the muscles for three days before a
three-day carbohydrate loading — the result is, theoretically,
a 100 per cent increase in endurance-type performance,
though there is an accompanying risk that the system can be
upset by the sudden change in normal habit and that this,
occurring immediately before a competition, could affect the
performance in the event.

Carbohydrates supply nearly all the energy for running
until you have progressed for half to three-quarters of an
hour, when the fat-burning mechanism switches in as an
energy source. Therefore, if you advance to marathon or
long-distance competition, bear in mind that the pre-
competition meal probably contributes little to your energy
needs during the event. You have to do the building much
sooner.

Studies also indicate that liquids are the best source of food and energy for competition events, dispelling the meat and potatoes notion, and that the fasting state, or one near it, may be most efficient for athletes. Liquid meals empty from the stomach fairly quickly, getting rid of that loaded feeling; they also help diaphragm action and make breathing easier.

Don't restrict your intake of water or other liquids during training or racing. It could lead to serious consequences, even fatal ones, as discussed earlier.

Normal diets contain an excessive amount of protein and it has been found that protein in excess quantity does not help muscle bulk but simply turns to expensive solid waste product.

Medical opinion now is that the eating of large quantities of carbohydrates is good for training athletes, because they use them, burn them up and, on the whole, show extremely low blood sugar counts.

Diet and hard training do not go together as a way of losing weight. The two should not be combined. If you diet and reduce your calory intake, the ability to replace those calories in terms of carbohydrates stored in muscles and liver will be reduced and your ability to perform will decrease substantially.

The worst thing you can do as a jogger is to starve or dehydrate yourself.

United States Air Force doctors Bruce C. Harger, James B. Miller and James C. Thompson published these tables in the *Journal of the American Medical Association* showing the calorific costs of running. They are worth studying by anyone adopting a jogging programme.

Table 1: Calories used per mile of running

Weight (pounds)	5:20	6:00	6:40	7:20	8:00	8:40	9:20	10:00	10:40
				Minutes pace per mile					
120	83	83	81	80	79	78	77	76	75
130	90	89	88	87	85	84	83	82	81
140	97	95	94	93	92	91	89	88	87
150	103	102	101	99	98	97	95	94	93
160	110	109	107	106	104	103	101	100	99
170	117	115	113	112	111	109	107	106	105
180	123	121	120	119	117	115	114	112	111
190	130	128	127	125	123	121	120	118	117
200	137	135	133	131	129	128	126	124	123
210	143	141	139	137	136	134	132	130	129
200	150	148	146	144	142	140	138	136	135

Note: expenditure of 3500 calories equals one-pound weight loss

Table 2: Calories used per minute

Weight (pounds)	5:20	6:00	6:40	7:20	8:00	8:40	9:20	10:00	10:40
				Minutes pace per mile					
120	15.6	13.8	12.1	10.9	9.9	9.0	8.3	7.6	7.0
130	16.9	14.8	13.2	11.8	10.7	9.7	8.9	8.1	7.6
140	18.1	15.9	14.1	12.6	11.5	10.5	9.6	8.8	8.1
150	19.4	17.0	15.1	13.5	12.3	11.2	10.2	9.4	8.7
160	20.6	18.1	16.1	14.5	13.0	11.8	10.9	10.1	9.3
170	21.9	19.2	17.0	15.3	13.8	12.7	11.5	10.6	9.8
180	23.1	20.2	18.0	16.2	14.6	13.3	12.2	11.2	10.4
190	24.2	21.3	19.0	17.0	15.4	14.0	12.9	11.8	10.9
200	25.6	22.4	19.9	17.9	16.2	14.8	13.5	12.4	11.5
210	26.9	23.6	20.9	18.7	17.0	15.5	14.1	13.0	12.1
220	28.1	24.7	21.9	19.6	17.8	16.2	14.8	13.6	12.6

Table 3: Calories used per hour

Weight (pounds)	5:20	6:00	6:40	7:20	8:00	8:40	9:20	10:00	10:40
				Minutes pace per mile					
120	936	828	726	654	594	540	498	456	420
130	1014	888	793	708	642	582	534	492	456
140	1086	954	846	756	690	630	576	528	486
150	1164	1020	906	810	738	672	712	564	522
160	1236	1086	966	870	780	708	654	600	558
170	1314	1152	1020	918	828	762	690	636	588
180	1386	1212	1080	972	876	798	732	672	624
190	1464	1278	1140	1020	924	840	774	708	654
200	1536	1344	1194	1074	972	883	810	744	690
210	1614	1416	1230	1122	1020	930	846	780	726
220	1686	1482	1314	1176	1068	972	888	816	756

19. Schedules

W E INCLUDE HERE some basic training schedules because, while jogging began as a keep-fit exercise and remains that primarily, inevitably an element of competition has crept in. Mass fun runs are now organised over distances from five kilometres up to 21-kilometre half-marathons; and a great many people who began jogging with no thought of doing any more than a turn or two around the local block have found themselves lured by their own improving physical condition into competing.

Many are ex-athletes taking up the sport again as veterans; many are total newcomers to competitive running. But their influence is so great that most organised running clubs and the events they conduct now provide veterans' divisions to cater for the new breed of runner.

Once you begin stepping out beyond elementary jogging and eyeing the fun runs, the middle-distance events and even the marathons within your reach, you need to prepare yourself properly and adequately to enjoy them as experiences in a new kind of living.

The schedules which follow simply set you up for the short fun run or for the longer ones up to the half-marathon. The first is suitable for all beginners, the second is designed for people who are into their second year or so of occasional competitive running and the third is for the more experienced people who have advanced to a point where they think more as runners than joggers.

The schedules are a guide only; it is not necessary or

desirable that you should slavishly follow each day's instructions. Since we are looking at competitive running only as an extension to jogging and not a stepping stone to the next Olympic Games, you should not hesitate to reduce the programme from day to day according to how you feel. For instance, it is better to run six windsprints and enjoy them than to force yourself through a dozen against your body's inclinations.

To help you to understand the schedules, the various components are:

Aerobic running — This is more than jogging but it must be strictly controlled. The speed should always be just below your maximum steady state, the pace at which you can comfortably run without exhausting yourself and creating an undesirable oxygen debt. A carefully regulated programme of aerobic running — training without straining — results in a progressive raising of the steady state and, of course, a consequential increase in the pace of your aerobic running. This is stamina training; other elements are added later in each schedule to provide anaerobic training, in which you deliberately exceed your maximum steady state for controlled periods and distances to further improve your steady state and to build up the capacity to withstand anaerobic exercise in which an oxygen debt is created.

Fartlek — Swedish for speed play, this involves running at various speeds over forest trails, parks and country at will. It incorporates aerobic and anaerobic running, usually according to the condition and capabilities of the runner on the day. Stride out here, sprint there, jog somewhere else, spring up a hill and so on.

Time trials — Give your body a certain exercise to do often enough and it becomes efficient at it. This is true of running over certain distances. The idea is to run trials at or under the distance you are training for at a speed close to your best but not enough to exhaust you.

Repetitions — These are usually used to develop the anaerobic capacity by varying the numbers run, the distance run, the times that each run takes and the intervals taken between them. Train as much as you feel like; don't rigidly follow the schedule. You run until the oxygen debt incurred makes you feel tired.

Relaxed fast running — As it suggests, simply striding out strongly over the suggested distance and then floating or jogging an equal or longer distance before the next stride out.

Windsprints — A series of sprints interspersed with floats to develop your recovery rate. Don't strain to become the fastest sprinter in the world.

Hill springing and steep hill or steps running — Both are vital for developing flexible, supple, powerful muscles and tendons from the ankles upwards. In the former, you spring up a fairly steep hill, driving off the toes and lifting the body as high as possible, landing on the toes and then driving upwards again. Your forward progress up the slope is minimal; the concentration is on full leg extension and lifting your body against gravity. The steep hill or steps running involves equally full flexion of the ankles at each step, high knee lift and you drive forward rather than upward with a full extension of the driving leg from toe to hip. Ideally, you need a flat area at the top of your hill for a recovery jog before you stride back down and repeat the exercise. If you also have a flat at the bottom, you can use this for sprints over varying distances up to, say, 50 metres. This can be quite a rigorous training session and should be preceded by and followed with a quiet jog of up to 15 minutes as should all other exercise sessions involving speed running.

Leg speed — another exercise that explains itself. Run up to the recommended distance with your concentration entirely on moving your legs as quickly as possible. Go for high knee lift, which means keeping your hips well forward, and don't worry about stride length.

FUN RUN

For 6 weeks: Monday — Jog 15 to 45 mins
Tuesday — Jog 30 to 60 mins
Wednesday — Jog 15 to 45 mins
Thursday — Jog 30 to 45 mins
Friday — Rest or jog 30 mins
Saturday — Jog 15 to 45 mins
Sunday — Jog 30 to 60 mins

For 4 weeks: Monday — Relaxed striding 100m x 4 to 6 times
Tuesday — Jog 30 to 60 mins
Wednesday — Time trial 3000m
Thursday — Jog 30 to 60 mins
Friday — Rest or jog 30 mins
Saturday — Time trial 5000m
Sunday — Jog 45 mins to 1½ hours
For 4 weeks: Monday — Relaxed striding 200m x 4 to 6 times
Tuesday — Jog 30 to 60 mins
Wednesday — Time trial 3000m
Thursday — Easy fartlek running 30 to 45 mins
Friday — Rest or jog 30 mins
Saturday — Time trial 5000m
Sunday — Jog 1 to 1½ hours
For 4 weeks: Monday — Repetitions 800m x 2 to 4 times
Tuesday — Jog 30 to 60 mins
Wednesday — Time trial 3000m
Thursday — Easy fartlek running 30 to 45 mins
Friday — Rest or jog 30 mins
Saturday — Time trial 5000m or 10,000m (alternate
weekly)
Sunday — Jog 1 to 1½ hours
For 2 weeks: Monday — Repetitions 1500m x 2 or 3 times
Tuesday — Jog 30 to 60 mins
Wednesday — Time trial 5000m
Thursday — Fast relaxed running 100m x 4 to 8 times
Friday — Rest or jog 30 mins
Saturday — Time trial 5000m 1st week, 10,000m 2nd week
Sunday — Jog 1 to 1½ hours
For 1 week: Monday — Windsprints (100m every 200m) x 6 to 8 times
Tuesday — Jog 45 mins
Wednesday — Time trial 2000m
Thursday — Fast relaxed running 100m x 4 to 6 times
Friday — Rest or jog 30 mins
Saturday — Time trial 3000m
Sunday — Jog 45 to 60 mins
For 1 week: Monday — Fast relaxed running 100m x 6 to 8 times
Tuesday — Time trial 1000m
Wednesday — Jog 45 mins
Thursday — Jog 30 mins
Friday — Rest or jog 30 mins
Saturday — FUN RUN
Sunday — Jog 45 to 60 mins

10,000 METRES to HALF-MARATHON
(second year joggers)

For 6 weeks: Monday — Aerobic running 30 to 45 mins
Tuesday — Jog 60 mins
Wednesday — Aerobic hill running 30 to 45 mins
Thursday — Jog 60 mins
Friday — Easy fartlek 30 mins
Saturday — Aerobic hill running 45 mins
Sunday — Jog 1½ hours

For 4 weeks: Monday — Easy fartlek 30 to 45 mins
Tuesday — Aerobic 1 to 1½ hours
Wednesday — Time trial 5000m
Thursday — Aerobic 1 to 1½ hours
Friday — Easy fartlek 30 mins
Saturday — Time trial 10,000m
Sunday — Jog 1½ hours

For 4 weeks: Monday — Leg speed running 100m x 6 to 8 times
Tuesday — Jog 1 to 1½ hours
Wednesday — Hill springing and steep hill or steps
running 30 to 45 mins
Thursday — Jog 1 to 1½ hours
Friday — Leg speed running 100m x 6 to 8 times
Saturday — Hill springing and steep hills or steps
running 30 to 45 mins
Sunday — Jog 1½ hours or more

For 4 weeks: Monday — Repetitions 400m x 6 to 10 times
Tuesday — Jog 1 to 1½ hours
Wednesday — Easy fartlek 45 mins
Thursday — Repetitions 200m x 8 to 12 times
Friday — Fast relaxed running 100m x 6 to 10 times
Saturday — Time trial 5000m
Sunday — Jog 1½ hours or more

For 4 weeks: Monday — Windsprints (100m every 200m) x 6 to 8 times
Tuesday — Jog 1½ hours
Wednesday — Time trial 3000m
Thursday — Easy fartlek 30 mins
Friday — Fast relaxed running 100m x 6 to 8 times
Saturday — Race or time trial 5000m
Sunday — Jog 1 hour or more

For 1 week: Monday — Windsprints (45m every 100m) x 8 to 12 times
             Tuesday — Easy fartlek 30 mins
             Wednesday — Time trial 5000m
             Thursday — Fast relaxed running 100m x 6 times
             Friday — Jog 30 mins
             Saturday — Race 1500m
             Sunday — Jog 1 hour
For 1 week: Monday — Windsprints (45m every 100m) x 10 times
             Tuesday — Fast relaxed running 100m x 6 to 8 times
             Wednesday — Time trial 800m
             Thursday — Jog 45 mins
             Friday — Jog 30 mins
             Saturday — First important race
             Sunday — Jog 1 hour or more
Continuation
of racing: Monday — Relaxed striding 200m x 6 times
             Tuesday — Easy fartlek 30 to 45 mins
             Wednesday — Time trial 3000m at ¾ effort
             Thursday — Jog 45 mins
             Friday — Jog 30 mins
             Saturday — Race
             Sunday — Jog 1 hour or more

10,000 METRES to HALF-MARATHON
(experienced joggers)

For 6 weeks: Monday — Aerobic running 45 to 60 mins
Tuesday — Jog 1½ hours
Wednesday — Aerobic hill running 45 mins
Thursday — Jog 1½ hours
Friday — Easy fartlek 30 mins
Saturday — Aerobic hill running 60 mins
Sunday — Jog 1½ hours or more

For 4 weeks: Monday — Easy fartlek 45 to 60 mins
Tuesday — Aerobic running 1½ hours
Wednesday — Time trial 5000m
Thursday — Aerobic running 1½ hours
Friday — Easy fartlek 45 mins
Saturday — Time trial 10,000m
Sunday — Jog 1½ hours or more

For 4 weeks: Monday — Leg speed running 100m x 8 to 10 times
Tuesday — Jog 1½ hours
Wednesday — Hill springing and steep hill or steps running 45 mins
Thursday — Jog 1½ hours
Friday — Leg speed running 100m x 8 to 10 times
Saturday — Hill springing and steep hill or steps running 45 to 60 mins
Sunday — Jog 1½ hours or more

For 4 weeks: Monday — Repetitions 400m x 8 to 12 times
Tuesday — Jog 1½ hours
Wednesday — Easy fartlek 45 to 60 mins
Thursday — Repetitions 200m x 10 to 15 times
Friday — Fast relaxed running 100m x 8 to 10 times
Saturday — Time trial 5000m
Sunday — Jog 1½ hours or more

For 4 weeks: Monday — Windsprints (100m every 200m) x 8 to 10 times
Tuesday — Jog 1½ hours
Wednesday — Time trial 3000m
Thursday — Easy fartlek 45 mins
Friday — Fast relaxed running 100m x 8 to 10 times
Saturday — Race or time trial 5000m
Sunday — Jog 1 hour or more

For 1 week: Monday — Windsprints (45m every 100m) x 12 to 16 times
Tuesday — Easy fartlek 45 mins
Wednesday — Time trial 5000m
Thursday — Fast relaxed running 100m x 6 to 8 times
Friday — Jog 30 mins
Saturday — Race 1500m
Sunday — Jog 1 hour

For 1 week: Monday — Windsprints (45m every 100m) x 12 times
Tuesday — Fast relaxed running 100m x 6 to 8 times
Wednesday — Time trial 800m
Thursday — Jog 45 mins
Friday — Jog 30 mins
Saturday — First important race
Sunday — Jog 1½ hours

Continuation of racing: Monday — Relaxed striding 200m x 6 times
Tuesday — Easy fartlek 45 mins
Wednesday — Time trial 3000m at ¾ effort
Thursday — Jog 45 mins
Friday — Jog 30 mins
Saturday — Race
Sunday — Jog 1½ hours